MRI Optimization

MRI Optimization
A Hands-on Approach

Peggy Woodward, B.S., R.T. (R)(MR)

Peggy Woodward & Associates
Partner, GPW Medical Imaging Consultants
San Francisco, California

William W. Orrison Jr., M.D.

New Mexico Institute of Neuroimaging
Professor of Radiology
Assistant Professor of Neurology
University of New Mexico School of Medicine
    and Albuquerque Veterans Administration Medical Center
Albuquerque, New Mexico

McGraw-Hill
Health Professions Division

New York   St. Louis   San Francisco   Auckland   Bogotá   Caracas   Lisbon   London   Madrid
Mexico City   Milan   Montreal   New Delhi   San Juan   Singapore   Sydney   Tokyo   Toronto

McGraw-Hill

A Division of The **McGraw·Hill** *Companies*

MRI OPTIMIZATION

1234567890   DOCDOC   9876

ISBN 0-07-071801-6

This book was set in Times Roman by Digitype.
The editors were James T. Morgan and Muza Navrozov.
The production supervisor was Richard Ruzycka.
The cover was designed by Michael Troller and Matthew Dvorozniak.
The index was prepared by Alexandra Nickerson.
R.R. Donnelley & Sons was printer and binder.

This book is printed on recycled, acid-free paper.

Library of Congress Cataloging-in-Publication Data

Woodward, Peggy.
    MRI optimization : a hands-on approach   /   Peggy Woodward, William W. Orrison Jr.
      p.   cm.
    Includes bibliographical references and index.
    ISBN 0-07-071801-6
    1. Magnetic resonance imaging.   I. Orrison, William W.
  II. Title.
    [DNLM: 1. Magnetic Resonance Imaging—methods.   WN 185W878m 1997]
  RC78.7.N83W66   1997
  616.071548—dc20
  DNLM/DLC
  for Library of Congress

Contents

Part III   *Practical Imaging*

Preface

Magnetic resonance imaging (MRI) represents one of the most significant developments in modern medicine. Never before in the history of medicine have health care providers been able to visualize with such detail the anatomy and pathology that exist within each of us. The magnetic resonance technologist is the keeper of the keys to this phenomenal resource. She or he can literally open the door to the human body in ways that could never have been dreamed of just a decade or two ago. The direction that this technology takes will be determined to a large extent by the technologists who interact on a daily basis with this most amazing of medical imaging tools. The technologists' "need to know" is perhaps greater in this field of imaging than in any other. The number of variables available to the operator of a modern magnetic resonance scanner can be mind-boggling. Yet with no fanfare or glory, the MRI technologist toils on in an arena that is ever changing and ever challenging. This is both the wonder and the horror of the job. This book attempts to make the work of the MRI technologist both more enjoyable and more effective.

It is the goal of *MRI Optimization: A Hands-on Approach* to describe in detail the factors that affect image quality and how the successful manipulation of scan parameters can produce unsurpassed image quality. We begin in Part I by discussing the factors that contribute to the production of the MR image. In every chapter, we describe how each circumstance can affect the final image and what can be done to counter any detrimental conditions.

In Part II, the chapters focus on special techniques that can be used to optimize image quality, from fast scan techniques to artifact-suppression methods. The techniques are described in enough detail to provide the operator with the intellectual tools needed to select the proper imaging technique for challenges encountered.

Part III is devoted to the practical aspect of individual structures of the human body. Each chapter begins with a review of the anatomy and pathology most often seen in that particular structure. This review is supported by pulse sequence selections and image optimization techniques.

MRI is both the present and the future of medical imaging, and the MRI technologist shares this vantage point. This book is a guide intended to provide the MRI technologist with the essentials needed to successfully manipulate pulse sequences according to any special circumstances encountered. We hope it will help the MRI technologists provide better patient care with less effort and more impressive results.

Without the dedicated efforts of key individuals, the completion of this book would not have been possible. We wish to acknowledge and extend our sincerest appreciation to Sheila Mulligan-Webb, who steadfastly edited the manuscripts; John A. Sanders, Ph.D., for his technical review; Carol Garner for her anatomic artwork; David Kramer, Ph.D., for his technical input; Nancy Correa and Diane Clark for generating images after hours from their MRI site at Queen of the Valley Hospital in Napa, California; Mary Espinosa, R.N., for her support in organizing the MR images; Jim Janis for his photography efforts; and Michael Troller of Michael Troller Design for his book cover scheme. Thanks are also in order and are expressed for images provided by Toshiba America Medical Systems, Inc., LUNAR Corporation, and Open MRI of Phoenix. Last, this book would not have been conceived without the contribution of creative ideas by all those MRI technologists who have crossed our paths. Thank you!

MRI Optimization

Part *I*

Factors that Affect Image Quality

1

The Patient

The patient is an often forgotten subject in discussions of image quality. In fact, the patient's body habitus, clinical status, tendency to show claustrophobic reactions in the magnet, and ability to tolerate the time component of the procedure are major factors contributing to the quality of the final images.

Body Habitus

The body habitus of the patient has a tremendous impact on our ability to obtain images that are of good diagnostic quality. Because nuclear magnetic resonance (NMR) is based on the interaction of radio-frequency (RF) photons with nuclei, the more nuclei per unit volume, the higher the RF absorption and the greater the potential signal return. In a patient who is obese, the common perception is that since lipids contain a relatively large number of hydrogen protons, signal will be maximum. However, proton density in soft tissue is quite uniform at a given temperature, and so the factor that affects signal-to-noise ratio (SNR) is the number of nuclei per voxel volume. In an obese person, there may in fact be less hydrogen contained in a given voxel volume than that found in the same voxel volume in a nonobese patient. Essentially, the tissue components are spread throughout a larger total area on an obese patient. Signal production can be hampered by spin-spin interactions between hydrogen and other tissue components as well.

In addition, there is more potential for motion artifacts from the tissues that are not constrained. The net result may be a degradation of image quality. In contrast, if the patient is extremely thin, loading of the coil may not occur, so that transmit power and receiver gain may be unobtainable or suboptimal. This may result in inability to collect images or in clipping errors resulting from lack of return signal. In either case, the assessment of the patient's body habitus is paramount in the selection of techniques that will effectively produce the image quality we desire.

If the body girth touches the inside facade of the magnet, coupling between the coil of the magnet and the patient's body may occur, resulting in image artifacts. Coupling in magnetic resonance imaging (MRI) is the result of an interaction between the patient and the magnetic imaging system; this can interfere with the collection of data. Coupling may also diminish the system's ability to select the correct RF power and receiver gain during the prescan process, which may inhibit optimal imaging. In addition, if the imaged areas exceed any field of view (FOV) (this would include the FOV of the magnet, RF transmit coil, gradient coil, RF receive coil, and the operator-selected FOV), aliasing or wraparound artifact can occur. This is especially evident in coronal imaging of the body where the diameter at the widest point, usually the hips or shoulders, is greater than the FOV of the gradient coil system, even if we have selected an acquisition FOV that we think will accommodate the patient's body. If the patient is quite large and touches the side walls of the magnet, coupling results, producing an "hourglass" appearance of the imaged volume where it has exceeded the homogeneous portion of the main magnetic field, as shown in Fig. 1-1.

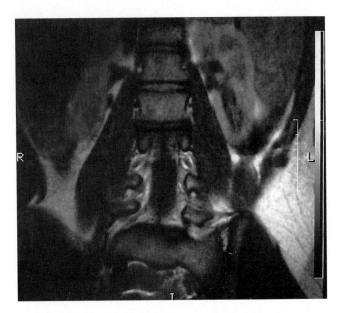

Figure 1-1 Image of coronal "hourglass" artifact.

Table 1-1 identifies methods that can be used to help provide adequate imaging of the very large or very small patient.

The patient may have a physical restriction, such as severe kyphosis, which limits the ability to recline supine on the table. MR imaging is unique in that scanning can be accomplished with the patient lying in any orientation. This includes placing the patient in a decubitus or semioblique position on the table. Therefore, physical limitations should not prevent the technologist from attempting to perform the exam. The patient can be propped in a position that will allow tolerance of the procedure, making it possible to finish the exam. This can be accomplished by using foam sponges placed about the patient as props. Many sites keep a supply of foam sponges of various sizes and shapes for this very purpose.

When adjusting the patient's position in the scanner using sponges, two important concepts must be appreciated:

- The sponges must be made of material that will not affect the magnetic field or produce RF interference. It

may be necessary to perform quick scans on sponges intended for use in the MR suite to assess MR compatibility.

- If the patient's condition necessitates placing him or her in a decubitus position, remember that most scanners associate anatomic position with the X-Y-Z axes of the magnet (see Table 1-2), so that selecting a coronal imaging plane will now result in a sagittal scan and vice versa. Transaxial imaging will always remain the same, but can be right left reversed. Newer patient positioners use information such as "head first, supine" to adjust for these changes.

TABLE 1-1 PATIENT BODY HABITUS IMAGING TIPS

Very Large

Use the smallest coil allowable for the body part.

Use sponges or padding between the body part and the transmit/receive coil.

Use sponges or pads to prevent direct contact of the body part with the magnet facade.

Use compression bands to restrict tissue movement, especially if imaging the torso.

Use the shortest scan times possible.

Consider imaging the patient in a prone position to minimize respiration and tissue movement.

Use scan parameters resulting in larger voxel volumes (i.e., thick slice and larger pixel dimension).

Use antialiasing techniques to minimize wraparound artifact.

Choose a FOV that adequately covers the area of interest.

Very Small

Use the smallest coil available for the body part.

Improve the efficiency of the imaging coil (called the Q of the coil) by using sufficient padding around the body part to help fill the coil.

Decrease the receive gain (RC) by several decibels, if the system allows this, to adjust for suboptimal loading of the coil.

TABLE 1-2 PATIENT ORIENTATION IN CONVENTIONAL MRI UNIT

Axis	Magnet Orientation	Anatomic Orientation	Imaging Plane
X	Across bore	Left-right	Sagittal
Y	Vertical	Anterior-posterior	Coronal
Z	Through bore	Head-foot	Transaxial

Note: Supine or prone, head first or feet first.

Clinical Status

The clinical status of a patient can yield many clues to whether the technologist will be able to obtain diagnostic information successfully. Generally, patients are referred to the imaging center along with a clinical history that is relevant to the exam ordered—for example, an order for a brain scan on a patient who has a "four-week history of occipital headaches and visual disturbances." Frequently, however, if a patient does not fit the appearance of a candidate for MR imaging, the result is cancellation of the test rather than an attempt to image the patient.

Imaging Patients with Motor Function Disturbances

Parkinsonism is the name given to a disturbance of motor function. Along with the typical symptoms of an expressionless face, stooped posture, slowness of voluntary movement, and a progressively shortened, accelerated gait, a characteristic tremor may also be present. Often all that is required in imaging these patients are support devices such as sponges under the offending extremities. With the extremities resting on sponges, the body is not striving to perform the motor function of holding the body part in place; thus the tremor may be significantly reduced and imaging may commence.

Claustrophobia

It is said that one out of four humans has claustrophobic tendencies. The patient may not realize it until confronted with the MRI scanner. The scheduling personnel attempt to deal with this issue by asking the potential patient about claustrophobia before he or she comes to the imaging center. In many cases, attempting to explain the procedure may in fact result in the patient's being talked into the condition.

A better approach may be to describe the procedure in fairly accurate detail, explaining that the patient is accessible by the technologist at any time should she or he need assistance. By tactfully describing the appearance of the scanner ("it is a large, long, cylindrical-shaped instrument which you will be lying in—we'll turn on the fan and light"), the noise it will make ("we'll give you earplugs, or, if you wish, you can bring a tape or CD of your favorite music and we will be happy to play it for you during the procedure"), the amount of time it will require to image the area of interest ("we'll perform about three to five different scans on you that will take between 30 s and 15 min each"), and what is expected ("we'll make you as comfortable as possible because you will need to hold

very still during the actual imaging time"), the site can defuse a lot of preconceived fears about the MR imaging process prior to patient arrival. The scheduler may then ask the patient if he or she expects to have any problems with the procedure. In some instances, it may be advantageous to have the potential patient come to observe the scanner prior to being scheduled.

A patient who is truly claustrophobic, as ascertained by previous experience with MRI, will virtually always let the imaging site know of this condition. In most cases there is no prior experience, however, and so the site must glean the information from the patient by asking questions relevant to the issue. If a patient is extremely large, he or she may exhibit claustrophobic tendencies, and so it is always a good idea to ask a patient's approximate height and weight. If the patient has had problems with diagnostic imaging procedures such as CT or nuclear medicine, she or he may also have claustrophobic tendencies with MRI. Knowing this before the scan day arrives allows both the patient and the imaging site to be prepared for circumstances that might hinder the imaging process.

Dementia, Pediatrics, and Uncooperative Patients

Patients in these groups, although highly variable and unlike one another, are similar in terms of the results we may obtain with the imaging procedure. Each group is difficult for different reasons; however, most of these patients can be imaged.

Often, the more you attempt to restrain a patient, the greater the fighting and the worse the images. In many cases, the demented patient and the pediatric patient can be treated the same way, using tenderness and coddling, much as you would treat your own loved ones. Often the patient can be talked through the procedure by using words of kindness throughout or by making a game of the procedure. Just hearing the voice of someone familiar during the scan can alleviate fear and confusion, rendering the patient more cooperative.

In the claustrophobic, demented, or uncooperative patient and the pediatric patient, open-bore magnets help to eliminate most of the anxieties associated with the MR imaging system. The patient can see and can be seen. However, that is not an operator-selectable parameter. MRI companies that manufacture this type of equipment can be contacted for the location of these imaging systems.

There are many methods that can be used to image the difficult patient. They are listed in Table 1-3. Sedation is purposely listed last, as all nonsedative techniques that are available should be attempted prior to giving a chemical sedative.

TABLE 1-3 TIPS FOR IMAGING THE DIFFICULT PATIENT

Technique	Advantages	Disadvantages
Change patient position: feet first, decubitus or oblique position, prone.	Enhances patient comfort; less potential for motion.	Adjustment of the selected plane of orientation may be necessary when using unconventional positioning.
"Sweet-talk" the patient into having the scan.	Scan can be done without sedation.	May increase total scan time.
Use fast scanning techniques, i.e., FSE, half-acquisition-imaging, gradient echo imaging, etc.	Reduces scan time without compromising image contrast; can significantly reduce flow artifacts.	Some techniques may be more sensitive to magnetic susceptibility effects (i.e., GRE) or truncation artifacts (i.e., FSE).
Scan patient at end of day.	Can spend more time with patient; reduces stress and anxiety of operator and patient.	May require personnel to work after hours.
Sleep deprivation	Physiologic sedation without the side effects of chemical sedation.	Hard on parents or other care givers.
Sedation	Reduces patient motion and physiologic motion.	Risks associated with chemical-induced sedation; patient monitoring required.

Patient Preparation

Adequate patient preparation includes the following:

- Explaining the procedure in detail to the patient
- Screening the patient for contraindications to MRI
- Providing the patient with MRI-compatible clothing
- Making the patient as comfortable as possible

In spite of the fact that metallic and RF artifacts are well documented in the field of MRI, sites continue to scan patients in clothing and jewelry that conceivably may produce these artifacts. In addition, scan doors may be left open during the imaging procedure—a perfect conduit for RF interference. These types of artifacts degrade image quality by lowering the SNR and causing distortions to the image. They delay imaging procedures by causing repeat scans to be performed. They may in fact create credibility issues at an imaging site if the site becomes notorious in the medical community for producing suboptimal images.

Clothing can contain ferromagnetic (iron, cobalt, nickel) or paramagnetic (titanium, platinum) materials, such as labels that contain ferromagnetic stainless steel thread. Many shoes contain metal in the soles. This can result in metallic artifacts that degrade image quality. Jewelry commonly contains an alloy for strength and durability that often is made of ferromagnetic (nickel) or paramagnetic (titanium) substances. It takes only a minimal amount of metal to result in decreased SNR values—approximately one gram, or roughly the amount of metal in the zipper of a pair of jeans or an underwire bra (see Fig. 1-2).

There is a common misconception that if the article of clothing is not within the FOV being imaged, there will be no loss of image quality. However, if one recalls the basic principles of magnets and magnetism, when ferromagnetics are used to shim or configure the homogeneous magnetic field, any additional metal that is brought into the magnetic environment can produce the same result. In addition, if a magnet is strong enough to cause deflection of a metallic object at the bore of the magnet or even within the 5-gauss line, it can certainly cause disruption toward the center of the magnet. The basic rule of thumb is that any change in magnetic field homogeneity can adversely affect image quality.

RF artifacts can result from any interference to the resonant frequency by a different radio frequency. Clothing that contains wool or nylon can produce static electricity, resulting in RF artifacts, known as "herringbone." This is especially true in dry environments. The static electricity created by the material actually interferes with the RF being used to produce the images. The appearance of this artifact is not unlike that of other types of RF interference.

It is essential to adequately evaluate patient clothing for potential artifact-producing materials or, better yet, provide the patient with a 100 percent cotton garment that is comfortable and that has been proven MR-compatible. This may involve scanning the garment to be used at the imaging site before signing with the linen company.

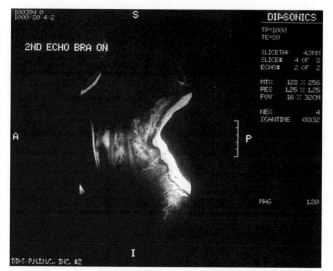

A

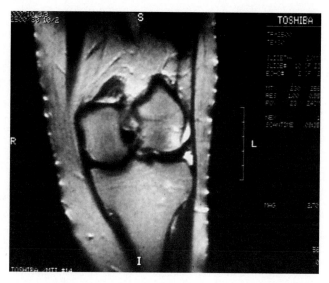

Figure 1-3   Image of knee with lotion artifacts.

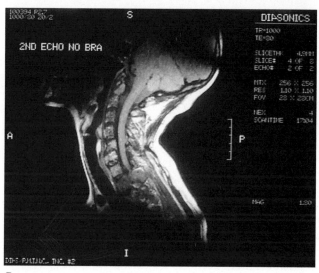

B

Figure 1-2   Cervical spine with (*A*) and without (*B*) brassiere present.

Other patient-related articles that have been shown to contribute to artifacts and a loss of image quality are as follows:

- Hairpins
- Safety pins
- Eyeglasses

- Wristwatches
- Dental devices
- Hearing aids
- Brassieres
- Boxer shorts with snaps
- Sanitary napkin belts
- Heavily applied makeup (mascara, eye shadow, rouge)
- Baby oil
- Mousse or excessive hair gels and sprays
- Self-tanning lotions

To eliminate the introduction of articles that can adversely affect image quality, it is recommended that the patient be scanned only in clothing issued by the site that has been proven MRI-compatible. All jewelry should be removed. Excessive makeup, hair gels, and lotions should be removed from the intended imaging region (see Fig. 1-3).

Image optimization begins with the conscientious attitude of the imaging personnel during patient preparation. The time it takes to prepare the patient for the procedure is inconsequential when compared to the deleterious effects on image quality associated with poor imaging techniques.

2

Time

The amount of time spent scanning is proportional to the signal-to-noise ratio (SNR) of the image. However, one cannot scan forever. In this chapter, we discuss the impositions of time on the quality of the examination. We introduce an equation that demonstrates the relationship between the time of an examination and those parameters that directly contribute to it.

Scan time for 2DFT and 3DFT imaging is related to three main operator-dependent scan parameter selections, with an additional parameter contributing to the 3DFT scan time equation. The basic parameters are repetition time (TR), number of phase-encode steps in the matrix (#PE), and number of averages or acquisitions (NA or N_{acq}). Because of the concept of 3DFT imaging, the number of slices (NS) is included in the formula for 3DFT imaging time. Any increase in these scan-time parameters increases scan time in direct proportion. The formulas are as follows:

$$\text{2DFT Scan time (minutes)} = \frac{\text{TR (seconds)} \times \text{\#PE} \times \text{NA}}{60 \text{ (seconds)}}$$

$$\text{3DFT Scan time (minutes)} = \frac{\text{TR (seconds)} \times \text{\#PE} \times \text{NA} \times \text{NS}}{60 \text{ (seconds)}}$$

TR, #PE, and NA also affect signal-to-noise ratio and contrast. In addition, TR and NS have a relationship such that either can be affected by a change in the other. To optimize image quality, the technologist/radiologist team must ascertain the patient's condition, the clinical indication for the scan, and the patient's tolerance for the procedure before selecting scan parameters for the imaging sequences. All too often, protocols are selected that are routine and intended to work well for the general patient population. However, as our experience in radiology has shown, there is rarely an ideal patient, one who has the endurance and fortitude, body habitus, and willingness to cooperate for a procedure that requires the utmost collaboration with the imaging team. Evaluation and selection of each scan parameter that contributes to the scan-time equation as well as the determination of the necessary contrast, SNR, and resolution will ensure image quality that is optimal. We will now describe the effects on total image quality when changes in scan-time parameters are used to decrease imaging time.

TR is defined as the *time to repetition*. As technologists, we know it as "repetition time," and we know that this parameter controls the amount of time T1 growth is allowed before the RF is repeated. TR is usually selected based on clinical diagnostic requirements or the desired contrast. If T1 contrast is the focus, TR is chosen to be short so that tissues of various composition (i.e., fat, gray matter, white matter, CSF, muscle, liver, and spleen) which have different relaxation rates will recover to distinct levels on the T1 relaxation curve. In this way, maximal tissue contrast is guaranteed.

In addition to a short TR, a short TE is selected to minimize T2 contrast contribution.

Selecting a short TR decreases scan time in accordance with the scan-time formula. However, this manipulation of a scan parameter has distinct effects on contrast and signal. As can be seen in Fig. 2-1, the signal intensity drops when a TR that yields high T1 contrast is chosen. This is an expected consequence of using a short TR time because of the lower overall T1 growth for most tissues. Apparent proton density (PD) for all tissues is also decreased, since optimum PD can occur only if all tissues

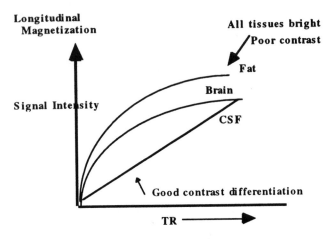

Figure 2-1 T1 growth curve.

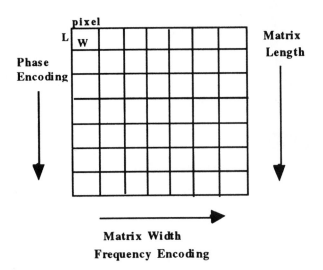

Figure 2-2 Matrix with *x* steps.

have been allowed maximum T1 growth. A decrease in TE also minimizes T2 contrast. This is necessary if the objective of the resultant image is T1 contrast.

A scan parameter that is often decreased to lower scan time is the number of steps in the phase-encode matrix, or #PE. A decreased #PE has a distinct effect on the resolution or detail of the image and a concomitant effect on the SNR. The phase-encode process is used to read the echoes many times by slightly changing the conditions under which they are read. We accomplish this by applying gradient magnetic fields in the third dimension of our slice (the slice thickness is our first dimension; the second dimension is selected by using a frequency-encode gradient to determine the distribution of spins at specific frequencies). The phase-encode gradient is applied at varying gradient strengths for each collection of data (equal to one line of phase encode). Since the frequency spread is different for each line of data collected, the phase coherence is also different. The larger the PE gradient, the greater the variance in spin phases.[1] In addition, by collecting many lines of data at varying gradient strengths, the ability to discern these data improves.

Decreasing the number of PE steps decreases the ability to spatially resolve the image information. We commonly refer to this phenomenon as a *loss of detail*. Each voxel of information is larger for a unique field of view and therefore contains more signal-producing data; thus the SNR for each voxel is increased. For the entire image, however, the SNR is decreased owing to a lack of collected data lines. Since we know that signal and contrast are coactive, a change in the matrix will also have an effect on resultant contrast. This effect is a result of Fourier transform and the process by which signal-intensity values for each voxel are averaged and converted to a gray-scale value for the resultant pixel (recall that currently images are displayed as two-dimensional objects; therefore voxels must be converted to pixels for display purposes). The

larger the voxel, the less all tissue signals contained in that voxel will have a unique contrast. If a small pathologic object is contained in a large voxel, its signal-intensity value will be averaged with that of the surrounding normal tissue. Thus the resultant gray-scale value will not be specific to the normal or abnormal tissue within the voxel but will be some combination of both. Figures 2-2 and 2-3 depict the relationship of the number of phase-encode steps to pixel size for a specific FOV.

Another consequence of decreasing the number of PE steps is the potential for an increase in visible truncation artifact. Truncation artifact is related to PE steps by the frequency difference from row to row. If there are large differences in frequency from row to row, as is the case when using a smaller number of phase-encode steps,

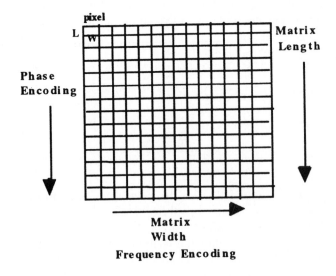

Figure 2-3 Matrix with 2× *x* steps.

the system sees a discontinuity in signal and mismaps that signal. This results in repetitious lines about the area of the discontinuity. Refer to Chap. 6 for a complete explanation of the truncation artifact.

The number of times the data are sampled without changing the phase-encoding gradient strength is known as the *number of acquisitions (N_{acq}) or averages* (NA). Increasing the NA increases scan time in proportion. In doing so, however, signal, which adds linearly, will increase, which will help to increase the overall SNR. Noise, which is statistical and random, will add incoherently, so that the actual effect on SNR is proportional to the square root of NA.

The greatest effect that lowering the NA has on the image is to decrease the SNR by the square-root factor and increase the propensity for visibility of motion artifacts because there is less averaging of random noise. Decreasing the number of times the data are collected has no effect on the contrast of the image.

The final scan parameter in the scan-time equation is related to 3DFT imaging techniques. In 3DFT imaging, separate slices are obtained by using a second phase-encode process. During fast Fourier transform, the slices are separated the same way resolution is defined in the phase-encode direction. Since phase encoding has a distinct effect on scan time, and since the number of slices necessary for a particular 3DFT sequence is related to phase encoding, an increase or decrease in the number of slices affects scan time proportionately. This becomes a drawback of 3D imaging, since the minimum scan time for a given TR is longer by a factor of the number of slice encodings.[2] As a result, most 3D imaging is performed with a gradient refocused echo technique using a short TR and flip angle.

Scan time can be shortened when performing 3DFT imaging by decreasing the number of slices. This has no effect on resolution, SNR, or contrast when conventional 3DFT imaging techniques are used. However, total coverage is decreased.

It should be noted that any factor that increases scan time has the disadvantage of creating the potential for an increase in motion artifacts. This is seen in Fig. 2-4A and B. Note the significant increase in anterior abdominal motion artifact seen in Fig. 2-4B.

Table 2-1 summarizes the advantages and disadvantages that changes in the scan-time parameters have on the resultant image.

Scan-time management is an important and sometimes frustrating concept in MR imaging. In an attempt to reduce artifacts caused by the intolerant patient, parameters that have a direct effect on scan time are adjusted. Many times the degradation of the resultant image as a result of lack of signal, resolution, averaging capabilities, or coverage is sufficient to far outweigh the benefits that would otherwise have been realized. The conscientious technologist must assess the ability of the patient to tolerate a procedure and manipulate scan parameters to obtain the best image possible in the least amount of scan time.

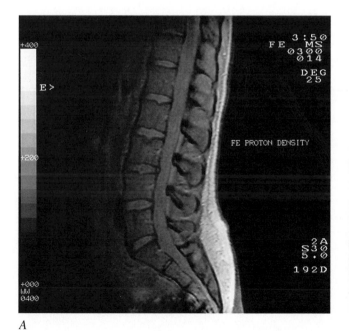

A

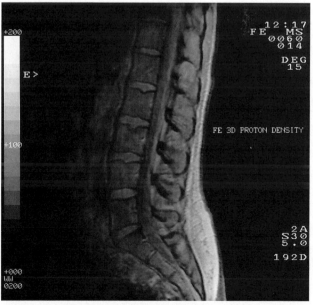

B

Figure 2-4   Motion artifacts in sagittal lumbar scan; 2DFT *(A)* and 3DFT *(B)*.

TABLE 2-1 SCAN-TIME PARAMETERS

Parameter	Change	Effect on ST	Advantage	Disadvantage
TR	Decrease	Decrease	Increase T1 contrast; decrease motion; decrease T2 contrast; decrease scan time	Decrease T1 growth; decrease SNR; decrease PD
Number of PE	Decrease	Decrease	Increase SNR/voxel; decrease motion; decrease scan time	Decrease overall SNR; increase truncation
Number of data sets (NA, N_{acq})	Decrease	Decrease	Decrease motion; decrease scan time	Decrease SNR by square root; decrease image averaging
Number of slices (3DFT only)	Decrease	Decrease	Decrease scan time	Decrease coverage

References

1. Schwartz GM: Relating the frequency to space: The fourier transform and gradient fields, in Woodward P, Freimarck R (eds): *MRI for Technologists*. New York: McGraw-Hill, 1995.

2. Sweitzer MC, Kramer DM: Standard MR pulse sequences: A closer look, in Woodward P, Freimarck R (eds): *MRI for Technologists*. New York: McGraw-Hill, 1995.

3

Contrast

In MRI, contrast is the difference in relative brightness between pixel values—the result of the signal intensity received from each voxel during the NMR experiment.[1] Contrast is inherent in tissues predominantly as a result of hydrogen proton concentration and the chemical bonding properties of this nuclear species with other tissue components. The result is variations in tissue relaxation rates which produce a particular signal intensity that is later assigned a unique gray-scale value during Fourier transform. It is the goal of MR imaging to elucidate that contrast without misrepresentation.

The graphic processor performs the primary calculation that separates the encoded signal into its individual frequency components. A gray-scale value between 1 and 256, depending on the signal intensity, will be assigned to individual pixels. The highest signal intensity will receive the brightest gray-scale value, while the lowest signal intensity receives the darkest value. The ability to differentiate pixels is related to how many gray-scale values are represented in the image. A wide range of gray-scale values representing the pixels will provide the least amount of contrast, whereas a limited number of gray-scale values will provide the highest contrast or the most blacks and whites. Figure 3-1 represents a pixel interpolation of a transaxial head image.

Factors Which Affect Contrast

The pixel intensity representing the content of each voxel within the tissue is determined by the relationship of the tissues to one another. This relationship includes hydrogen proton concentration and the chemical bonding properties within the tissue. The contrast of the resultant image depends on this relationship and how it is manipulated by the selection of particular scan parameters. These scan parameters include TR, TE (echo time), TI (time to inversion), flip angle, and pulse sequence type. When using fast scan techniques, ETL (echo train length), ETE (effective TE), and ETS (echo train spacing) play a role in contrast manipulation. In addition, T1 and T2 relaxation rates, flow, and contrast media are aspects of MRI that have a definitive relationship to contrast.

Pulse Sequence Selection

The type of pulse sequence selected will help to determine the TR, TE, flip angle, and TI to use. However, it is the clinical criteria and desired contrast that result in the selection of a unique pulse sequence which, when combined with patient tolerance for the procedure, defines the scan parameters chosen. Each of the scan parameters—TR, TE, flip angle, and/or T1—will affect the contrast perceived in the final image. They must be chosen with care.

There are three main types of pulse sequence from which the MRI technologist and radiologist may choose. They are garden-variety pulse sequences that have been used since the inception of MR technology: spin echo (SE), gradient echo (GRE, FE), and inversion recovery (IR). Using these basic sequences, researchers have developed many different hybrids or modifications, each with its own specific function. Since many researchers are affiliated with specific manufacturers of MR equipment, each company has its own name for versions of the norm.

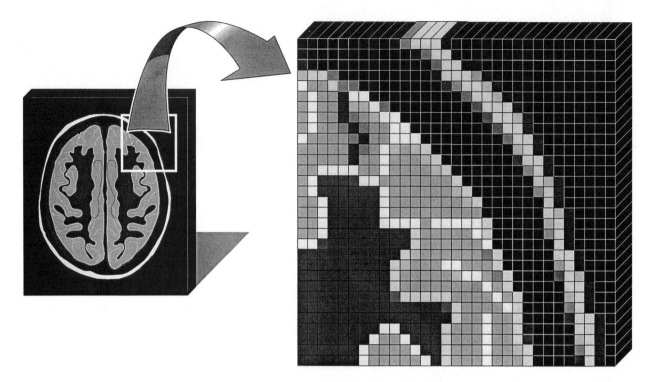

Figure 3-1   Pixel interpolation of a transaxial head image.

Most basic renditions of spin echo and gradient echo sequences can be manipulated to result in images with T1 or T2 contrast. In the SE sequence, the radio-frequency (RF) power level is calibrated to cause a transfer of the net magnetic vector at a 90° angle. In addition, a rephasing pulse using a 180° flip is used. The T1 relaxation time is related to recovery from the 90° flip. By varying the TR and TE, the sequence can be used to highlight T1 or T2 contrast, or merely to observe spin density.

If the magnetic vector representing the tissue is rotated less than 90°, it will return to equilibrium at a faster rate. The effect is as if T1 time were shorter. This is the phenomenon behind most gradient echo imaging techniques. The sequence is further modified from traditional SE techniques by the use of a reversal of the readout gradient to form the echo. The use of a lower FA allows the selection of a shorter TR, which results in a shortened scan time. Using gradient echo imaging techniques, one can adjust the TR, TE, and FA to provide contrast similar to that seen using conventional SE techniques; that is, T1 and T2 contrast as well as proton density images. Gradient echo sequences are used to obtain images that have contrast similar to that seen when using long TR times.

Inversion recovery pulse sequences generally are limited to T1 contrast development, with or without fat suppression. An RF pulse using a flip angle of 180° rotates the magnetic vector into the longitudinal plane, but in the opposite orientation. Since signal must be collected perpendicular to the magnetic field, the vector then must be rotated by 90°, where data can then be sampled. The time

between the initial 180° RF pulse and the subsequent 90° is called the *time to invert,* or TI time. This parameter must be selected by the operator as the contrast control factor of IR imaging.

Repetition Time (TR)

TR is the time interval between the RF at the beginning of a pulse sequence and at the end of the pulse sequence for the same slice. The perturbation of the longitudinally magnetized vector by the resonant frequency forces the vector into the transverse plane. During this time interval, T2 relaxation (loss of phase coherence) is occurring. However, in the scheme of things, this uses a relatively small part of the total TR. Figure 3-2 shows a graphic depiction of TR in a typical SE pulse sequence with two echoes.

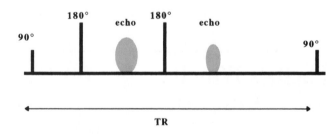

Figure 3-2   Repetition time (TR); conventional two-echo SE pulse sequence diagram.

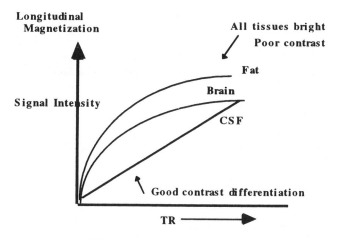

Figure 3-3   TI-contrast curve.

The additional time in the pulse sequence after the echo has been sampled is taken up by longitudinal regrowth and other processes involved in image formation. The longer the TR, the more *all* tissue vectors are allowed to recover, so that proton density for all tissues is maximal, resulting in high signal for all tissues but low contrast differentiation. When TR is chosen to be short, T1 tissue differentiation is maximal (see Fig. 3-3).

Since TR is related to T1 relaxation time, it must be chosen in accordance with its relationship with the field strength of the MR system. T1 relaxation time increases with increasing field strength. This is due in part to resistance and the added thermal motion of additional hydrogen atoms that have been affected by a stronger external magnetic field (see Fig. 3-4).

If T1 times are longer, the amount of time necessary for some component of longitudinal growth to occur will be longer. Protocol strategy is dictated by desired contrast, clinical appearance of the suspected pathology, and tolerance of the patient for being imaged, and is developed to take advantage of the unique relationship between T1 relaxation times and field strength.

Table 3-1 indicates general T1 relaxation times at different field strengths. It must be noted that T1 times will differ as a result of variations in the methods by which the data are collected at different research labs. Refer to the operating guides for the particular MR imaging system which you are using for a listing of appropriate T1 relaxation times.

When T1 contrast is desired, TR is selected to optimize T1 contrast by allowing some tissue vectors to recover longitudinal magnetization, thereby producing a strong signal, while other tissues are not allowed this recovery. In some cases, an image that depicts maximum concentration of hydrogen is requested. This is called a *proton density* image and is obtained in part by using a long TR. If T2 contrast is necessary, TR is chosen to be long to minimize T1 effects. Figure 3-5*A–C* represents TR changes at 0.35 T.

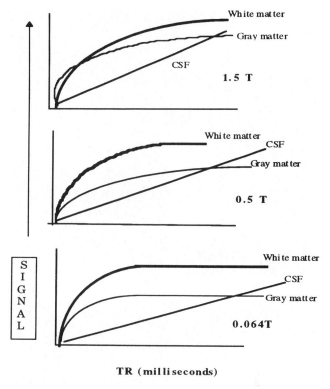

Figure 3-4   T1 contrast curves at low, mid, and high field.

Echo Time (TE)

TE is the time from the original RF pulse to the peak of its reemitted echo and is referred to as the time to echo (see Fig. 3-6). The signal information derived from the NMR experiment is sampled during this time.

Normally, data collection occurs very early in the pulse sequence; echo times usually range from 5 to 150 ms, whereas TR times are usually on the order of 30 to 5000 ms, depending on the pulse sequence being performed. Echo times are related to T2 loss of phase coherence, which is not field-strength-dependent; therefore, T2 tissue relaxation times are fairly consistent from one MR system to another. Table 3-2 gives mean T2 relaxation times for tissues.

TABLE 3-1 MEAN T1 RELAXATION TIMES IN MILLISECONDS

Tissue	0.15 T	0.5 T	1.0 T	1.5 T
Fat	150	215	220	250
Liver	250	323	420	490
White matter	300	539	680	783
Muscle	450	600	730	863
Spleen	400	554	680	778
Gray matter	475	656	809	917
CSF	2000	2000	2500	3000

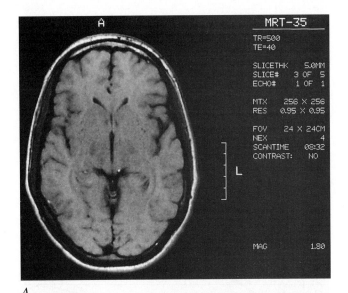

A

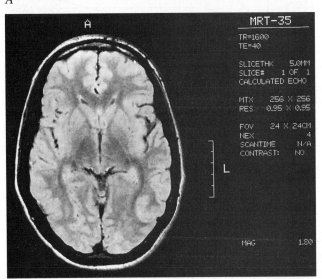

B

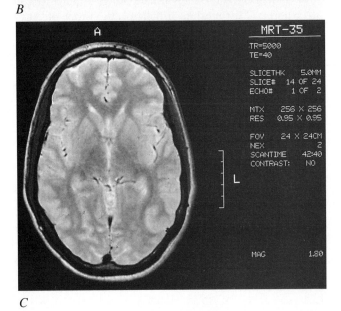

C

Figure 3-5 Transaxial brain. (*A*) TR 500 ms; (*B*) TR 1600 ms; (*C*) TR 5000 ms.

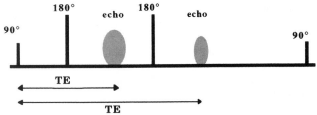

Figure 3-6 Echo time (TE); conventional two-echo SE pulse sequence diagram.

TE is chosen as a function of T2 decay. Spins in tissues that have short T2 decay times, such as tendons and ligaments, will lose their phase coherence rapidly, diminishing in signal intensity as a result. This is due to rapid fluctuations of the spins, which are random and chaotic and in a tight chemical bonding lattice. These structures are considered short T2 tissues because their energy is transferred readily from spin to spin, which causes the loss of phase coherence. Spins in tissues that are plentiful and are loosely bound do not exchange energy as readily and therefore maintain their phase relationship for a longer period of time. We call these tissues *long T2 tissues*. They are found in structures that contain simple fluid, such as the ventricular system, the orbits, and the urinary bladder. Of great importance to our protocol decision-making process is the fact that pathologic structures have long T2 tissue relaxation times by virtue of their increased hydrogen proton concentration. That is, because of the inflammatory response of the body to the disease or trauma, the response is initiated and loosely bound hydrogen concentrates in the area of the insult. Since we know where fluid-filled structures reside and that they will remain bright for a long time after RF perturbation, and we know that the signals from short T2 tissues decay fairly early in the pulse sequence, we can deduce that any structure that is bright in an area that should be dark may be due to pathology. Figure 3-7 shows the T2 decay curve for tissues.

The images represented in Fig. 3-8*A*, *B*, and *C* show the increase in T2 contrast with an increase in TE time.

TABLE 3-2 MEAN T2 RELAXATION TIMES IN MILLISECONDS

Tissue	T2, ms
Fat	85
Liver	43
White matter	90
Spleen	62
Gray matter	100
Muscle	47
CSF	1400

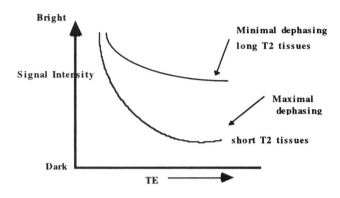

Figure 3-7 T2 tissue relaxation curve.

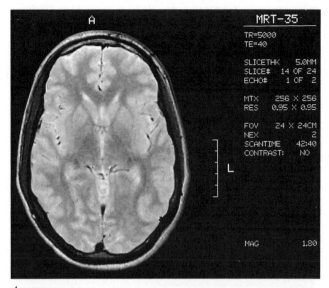

A

Time to Inversion (TI)

Time to inversion is essentially the T1 growth time factor allowed before an inverted vector is flipped into the transverse plane for subsequent data collection. The TI time is the contrast-controlling scan parameter used with inversion recovery (IR) pulse sequences and is chosen based on diagnostic tissue contrast requirements. If the tissue vector is crossing the transverse plane, also known as the null point of the signal, when data are sampled, the signal intensity of that tissue will be minimal. Figure 3-9 depicts this phenomenon.

When performing IR techniques such as STIR (short-TI inversion recovery) because of their fat-suppression capabilities, the TI is chosen so that it is approximately 69 percent of the T1 relaxation time of fat at the field strength at which the study is being performed. This ensures that the signal from fat will be minimal. When differentiating between tissues with fairly close T1 relaxation times, such as gray and white matter, the TI should be much longer in order to produce images with greater contrast between these CNS structures. The TI is determined by approximating the mean T1 relaxation values of the tissues being imaged and using that value. Figure 3-10A and B represents IR images using different TI values.

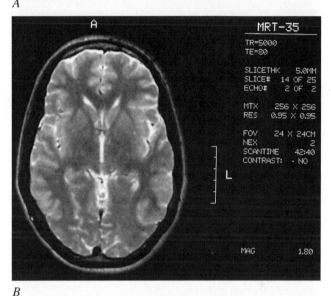

B

Flip Angle (FA)

The relaxation time of tissues is dependent on the magnetic fields encountered during the NMR experiment. It can be changed only if a magnetic field has changed. When sequences are used that allow the deliberate selection of a unique FA, such as gradient echo imaging or sequences requiring preparation pulses, relaxation rates become a function of that angle. For example, if the FA is chosen to be 45°, the tissue vector will recover longitudinal magnetization (T1 growth) more quickly than when using a conventional SE pulse sequence where the FA is 90°. The TR must be adjusted to accommodate this increased relaxation time. For this reason, gradient echo se-

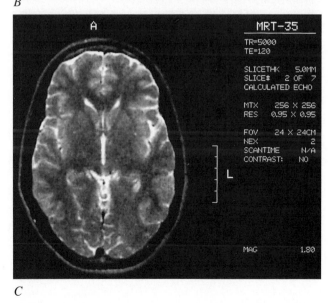

C

Figure 3-8 Transaxial brain. (A) TE 40 ms; (B) TE 80 ms; (C) TE 120 ms.

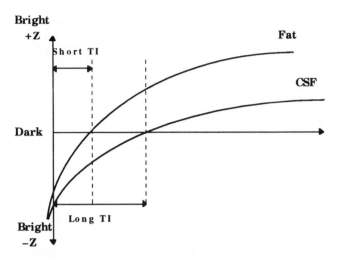

Figure 3-9   Effect of TI on signal intensity.

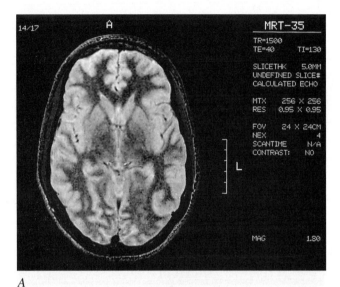

A

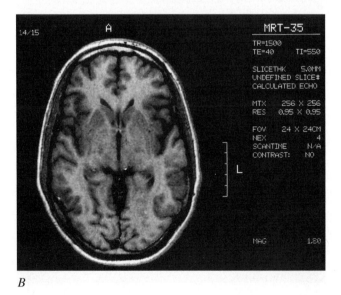

B

Figure 3-10   Transaxial brain. (*A*) TI 130 ms; (*B*) TI 550 ms.

quences can be accomplished at a faster rate than SE sequences. Image techniques using partial flip technology provide methods to obtain image contrast similar to that seen using long TR sequences (T2-weighted SE sequences) in shorter imaging times.

Figure 3-11*A–C* shows guides that can be used to predict a best-guess flip angle. Selection of flip angle is still a matter of experience, however, because T1 does not tell the whole story; there are still spin density and T2. In addition, contrast varies from system to system and from patient to patient. These guides are intended only as a reference in selecting approximate flip angles.

To use the graphs, select the TR value for the sequence from the TR values on the right. Identify from the left the SE TR that would normally yield the contrast you are trying to simulate (i.e., longest TR for high T2 contrast). Trace the curve associated with the TR to the horizontal line corresponding to the SE curve. Drop a vertical line to the best-guess FA.

The images seen in Fig. 3-12*A–C* represent FE techniques using different flip angles.

Effective TE (ETE), Echo Train Length (ETL), and Echo Train Spacing (ETS)

When performing fast scan sequences, such as fast SE, the effective TE, echo train length, and echo train spacing become important contrast factors. The effective TE (ETE) essentially describes the contrast observed on the final image. It is a mixture of all echoes collected in the echo train (refer to Chap. 7 for a complete description of fast scan sequences). Contrast is normally derived from the middle of k space. K space is the "information folder" in which data are placed during acquisition. Frequency information pertaining to contrast and signal is normally placed in the middle of k space, while the periphery of k space contributes to spatial resolution. The lines of k space are commonly known as the phase-encoding rows, which are made up of data samples or readout information; each row of data contains all the information necessary to create an image. Since the ETE is actually a mixture of all echoes collected during a fast SE sequence, it may appear to have more or less contrast depending on the length of the echo train and at what millisecond the first and last echoes are sampled. The shorter the echo times, the more contribution from T1 contrast. The farther out the echo times within the train, the more T2 contribution. In other words, in two sequences that use the same ETE but have different starting and ending echo times because of the specific pulse sequence design, the images can have different contrast.

The echo train length (ETL) describes the number of echoes collected during one repetition. The longer the ETL, the more possibility for T2 contribution, since which get averaged during Fourier transform, resulting in the assignment of an arbitrary gray-scale factor.

It is important to know the specific details of fast scan sequences on the MR imaging system which the operator is using. Choosing the correct fast scan parameters can provide optimum contrast on the final image.

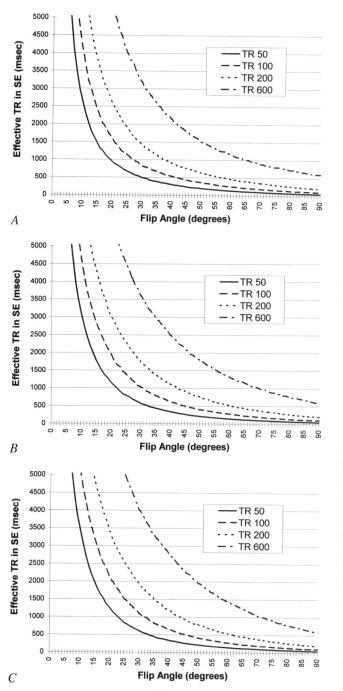

Figure 3-11 Best-guess flip angle at low (*A*), mid (*B*), and high (*C*) fields, respectively. *A.* Equivalent contrast TR at 0.064 T. *B.* Equivalent contrast TR at 0.5 T. *C.* Equivalent contrast TR at 1.5 T. Courtesy David Kramer, Ph.D.

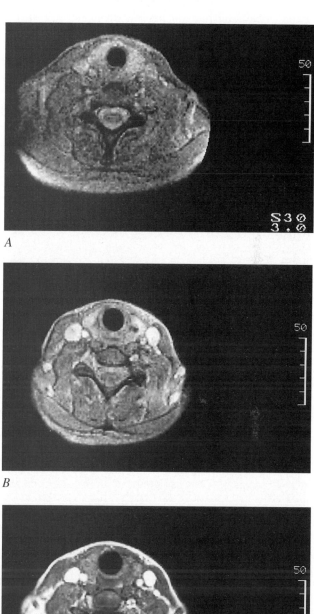

Figure 3-12 Three axial cervical images using flip angles of 6° (A), 10° (B), and 45° (C), respectively.

echoes contributing to the ETE are longer. In addition, if the echo train spacing (ETS) is increased with a long ETL, T2 contrast is even greater. However, an increase in ETS is also associated with the potential for an increase in blurring artifacts, which can ultimately reduce T2 contrast. This is due to a nonspecific frequency from the blurred edges being incorporated into voxel volumes

T1 and T2 Relaxation Times

Relaxation in MRI can be described as the time it takes the spin system to recover after being perturbed from equilibrium. Data sampling occurs in the form of echo collection based on desired contrast and can be adjusted to yield T1-weighted, T2-weighted, or proton-density images. The contrast of the image is determined by the unique relaxation rates of tissues, which depend on the magnetic susceptibility of nuclei within the tissue, external magnetic field inhomogeneities, and tissue type. In order to obtain images with contrast that promotes tissue differentiation, even at subtle levels, operators must have a concept of relaxation times for the magnetic field that is in use at their site. Figure 3-4 and Tables 3-1 and 3-2 identify T1 contrast curves at different field strengths and mean T1 and T2 relaxation times, respectively. It is important that protocol design incorporate the correct use of T1 relaxation times in determination of TR, since T1 is field-strength dependent.

Flow

Flow refers to the hydrogen that is in motion during the time of acquisition. It originates from blood, CSF, lymphatic, or bile. With respect to contrast, blood flow and CSF flow are the most confusing. They can be dark, bright, or any combination thereof. When consistent scan parameters are used, the expected appearance of normal blood vessels becomes familiar to the operator. However, when imaging parameters are arbitrary, the observed signals may become highly complex and difficult to explain.

Pulse sequence design as well as the physical characteristics of flow may have profound influences on the appearance of the vessel. The technical factors that affect the appearance of blood flow include the type of pulse sequence used (SE, GRE, or IR), TR, TE, and FA. Gradient moment nulling and presaturation techniques (see Chap. 12) and gated sequences also affect the appearance of blood flow. Even small changes in slice thickness, slice gap, slice order, and the number of slices can contribute to a variation in the contrast of the vessel. Variations in flow appearance between different MRI scanners may also exist, even when using identical scan parameters.

The physical characteristics of flow are related to flow dynamics. They include flow direction, velocity, acceleration, pulsatility, and vessel distribution. Patterns of flow, whether laminar, vortex, or turbulent, further influence the appearance of flow on MR images. Refer to Chap. 12 for a complete description of flow dynamics.

Several basic principles can be noted concerning the appearance of flow on MR images. They are summarized in Table 3-3. Those factors contributing to the appearance of signal within the vessel which are related to flow dynamics are the spin velocity and type of flow. When the velocity is slow and laminar, as in flow from the veins and CSF, spin signals tend to be collected when rephased, so that signal in the vessel is increased. This is true for spin echo and gradient echo techniques. However, when flowing spins are turbulent and rapid, as in arterial flow and certain vascular anomalies (AVM and aneurysms), dephasing occurs quickly, producing vascular signal loss on SE sequences.

Techniques used to compensate for artifacts produced by flowing spins have a distinct effect on observed vascular signal. Presaturation techniques applied outside the field of view effectively minimize any signal from moving spins by saturating the spins with RF before the signal is collected. If spins are not allowed to rephase, they will not produce a signal; hence, vascular structures will be dark. On the contrary, when gradient moment nulling techniques (flow compensation) are used, moving spins are forced to rephase, so that data collection results

TABLE 3-3 MR SIGNAL IN BLOOD VESSELS (BLOOD FLOW APPEARANCE ON MR IMAGES)

Increased	Decreased
Low velocity	High velocity
Laminar flow	Turbulent, vortex flow
Gradient moment nulling (flow comp)	Presaturation
Even-echo rephasing	Odd-echo rephasing
Acquisition with one slice	Multislice acquisition
Flow perpendicular to imaging plane	Flow parallel to plane of image
End slices closest to entry of blood flow	Slices furthest from flow entry
Gating	
Gadolinium	

Source: Elster AD: Flow phenomena and MR angiography, in *Questions and Answers in Magnetic Resonance Imaging*, St. Louis: Mosby, 1994. With permission.

in increased vascular signal. Some fast-flowing spins may still exhibit flow void since gradient sequence design to date has not been able to completely compensate for higher orders of moments (see Chap. 12).

Gated techniques may be used to improve the signal in all vessels. However, in many instances of cardiac gating, where multislice or multiphase acquisition is being performed, some images may display a signal void where data collection occurred during dephase of the moving spins.

Flow-related phenomena involving signal changes may be identified when performing symmetric SE multi-echo imaging techniques. An example would be when using echo trains such as TE 30, 60, 90, 120. Bright signal tends to be seen after the even echoes (60 and 120, or second and fourth echoes), whereas a signal void is noted following the odd echoes (30 and 90, or first and third echoes). This is known as even-echo rephasing and odd-echo rephasing, respectively. This phenomenon exists because of the fact that total phase shift increases quadratically with time for constant flow velocity through a constant gradient. There is also a 180° rephasing component that is used to calculate the total accumulated phase. For the first echo, an appreciable phase dispersion is noted in the flowing spins, resulting in decreased signal; this is the origin of odd-echo rephasing. The subsequent even echo has a significant total phase shift which calculates to 0. This means that the moving spins have recovered enough phase on the second echo to produce a bright signal (even-echo rephasing). The gradient responsible for this accentuation is the readout gradient. So, in fact, this phenomenon is commonly seen when flow is in the direction of the readout gradient.

The direction of flow within the imaging volume and the way in which it enters that volume (perpendicular versus parallel) also can affect signal and are exploited when performing MR vascular sequences (see Chap. 8). When fresh spins (unsaturated) enter the imaging volume, the signal of the spins is maximum. This is called *flow-related enhancement*; it is used in time-of-flight (TOF) technology. With movement through the volume, the flowing spins become saturated with every TR and lose their phase coherency; thus vascular signal diminishes. When performing 3DFT TOF sequences, whether the moving spins enter the volume parallel or perpendicular has little effect on signal. However, when using 2DFT TOF methods, where single-slice acquisition occurs, it is important that the slices be oriented perpendicular to blood flow for the best in-flow enhancement.

Finally, gadolinium injection generally increases the signal from all vessels. This is a result of the T1 and T2 shortening when using paramagnetic contrast media. The time necessary for GdDTPA to reduce its blood concentration by one-half is on the order of 100 min.[2] With time, the concentration of the drug in the blood will diminish;

however, until the point at which total elimination has occurred, the vessel will be bright in signal intensity. Even if a presaturation band is applied to suppress venous signal, flow dynamics dictate allowing some visualization of venous structures, especially those that are large, such as those found in the head.

Contrast Media

Many tissues possess biophysical properties that are quite similar, resulting in no appreciable difference in tissue contrast. Materials that alter intrinsic MR properties, proton spin density, or T1 and/or T2 relaxation times may be administered to enhance contrast differences. Positive contrast occurs when the media administered produce a brighter signal in the tissue of interest than without the media; negative contrast enhancement occurs when the tissue becomes darker after the administration of contrast media. Signal intensity will increase if proton density increases, T1 relaxation time decreases, or T2 relaxation time increases. Contrast agents have been developed to exploit these characteristics.[3]

The injectable contrast media most commonly used in MR imaging today consist of complexes of the element gadolinium (Gd), which is a paramagnetic metal. The observed signal from gadolinium is a result of the increased relaxation time of the tissues caused by the interaction of the *electrons* of Gd with the resonating protons of hydrogen. This causes the protons to recover to equilibrium more rapidly. The reduction of T1 results in an increase in signal intensity, while a reduction of T2 results in signal loss. Since the effect of T1 shortening predominates when a paramagnetic substance such as Gd is used, T1-weighted imaging techniques are used most commonly. However, it has been shown that when higher concentrations of Gd are injected, T2 reductions are more significant.[4] Therefore, with appropriate selection of pulse sequence parameters, T2 images may provide improved contrast enhancement when increased concentrations of Gd are employed.

Several MR contrast agents have been investigated for their improved T2 enhancement. Specifically, ferromagnetic, superparamagnetic, and susceptibility-enhancing agents may be used with T2-weighted imaging techniques to maximize T2 contrast.

MRI contrast is undoubtedly one of the most important factors contributing to image quality. Without contrast, subtle differences in tissues are difficult to establish. In most cases, contrast is indeed the factor that allows a diagnosis to be rendered. It is paramount that the operator of the MRI imaging system use knowledge and foresight in choosing scan parameters that contribute to contrast (see Table 3-4). Without contrast, the image becomes just another pretty picture.

TABLE 3-4 IMAGE PARAMETER EFFECT ON CONTRAST

Image Parameter	Action	Effect on Contrast
TR	Increase	Increases T2 contrast with high TE
		Decreases T1 contrast
	Decrease	Increases T1 contrast with low TE
		Decreases T2 contrast
TE	Increase	Increases T2 contrast with high TR
		Decreases T1 contrast
FA	Increase	Increases T1-like contrast
		Decreases T2° contrast
	Decrease	Increases T2° contrast
		Decreases T1 contrast
TI	Increase	Increases T1 contrast
	Decrease	Increases fat suppression
ETE	Increase	Increases T2 contrast
	Decrease	Depends on ETL and ETS
ETL	Increase	Increases contrast mix
	Decrease	Decreases contrast mix
ETS	Increase	Increases blurring artifact and may cause decrease in contrast
Pulse sequence	SE	T1 or T2 contrast depends on TR/TE
	FE	T1 or T2° contrast depends on TR/TE/FA
	IR	T1 contrast

References

1. Woodward P: Assessing the interaction of image sequence parameters, in Woodward P, Freimarck R (eds): *MRI for Technologists.* New York: McGraw-Hill, 1995.
2. Watson AD: MR contrast media, in Woodward P, Freimarck R (eds): *MRI for Technologists.* New York: McGraw-Hill, 1995.
3. Watson AD: MR contrast media, in Woodward P, Freimarck R (eds): *MRI for Technologists.* New York: McGraw-Hill, 1995.
4. Watson AD: MR contrast media, in Woodward P, Freimarck R (eds): *MRI for Technologists.* New York: McGraw-Hill, 1995.

4

Spatial Resolution

Spatial resolution is the degree to which the image exhibits clarity and definition. It is ultimately controlled by the size of individual tissue voxels. The slice thickness (ST), matrix (PE and RO), and field of view (FOV) have a direct relationship to voxel size, so that these parameters affect resolving power as well. In fact, voxel volume can be calculated by the following equations:

Voxel volume for 2DFT
$$= ST \times (FOV^{PE}/\#PE) \times (FOV^{RO}/\#RO) \qquad (4.1)$$

or

Voxel volume for 3DFT
$$= ST \times (FOV^{PE}/\#PE) \times (FOV^{RO}/\#RO) \times (FOV^{SS}/\#S) \qquad (4.2)$$

Following is a review of the definitions of the main factors contributing to spatial resolution.

Voxel   The smallest discrete three-dimensional object having length, width, and depth (see Fig. 4-1). The length and width are defined by pixel size, and the depth is determined by the slice thickness.

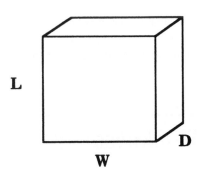

Figure 4-1   Voxel.

Pixel   The smallest discrete two-dimensional object having length and width; two dimensions of the initial voxel volume (see Fig. 4-2).

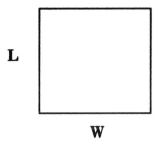

Figure 4-2   Pixel.

Matrix   An arrangement of voxels given a *Y* dimension or phase-encoding direction (PE) and an *X* dimension or frequency-encoding direction (RO) (see Fig. 4-3).

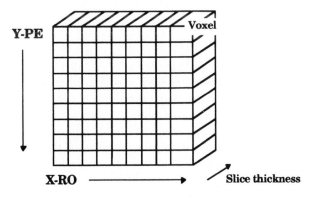

Figure 4-3   Matrix.

23

Slice thickness   The depth of the voxel or matrix.

Field of view (FOV)   The contour of the total tissue area (see Fig. 4-4).

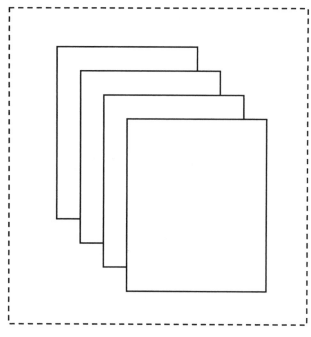

Figure 4-4   FOV.

Anatomic edge detail improves dramatically when voxel size is minimized. This is a result of the method by which image formation is accomplished. Images are created from signal averaging of tissue voxel elements. When voxel size is large, there is a higher degree of possibility that many diverse signals will be contained within the voxel. For example, when imaging an anatomic region that is small, such as the acoustic nerve, using a relatively large slice thickness and pixel size, the signal intensities of all surrounding tissues, no matter how diverse, will be included in the composite rendition of the voxel. Since these signals become a composite signal for pixel display, the resulting gray-scale value becomes ambiguous; that is, the displayed image intensity may not be specific to any one tissue element. This appears as a blurring of the image, resulting in a reduction in contrast differentiation and visibility of small structures. If the voxel size is small enough so that few different signal intensities are encoded within the voxel, spatial resolution as well as contrast improves because of the uniqueness of the signal. We commonly refer to this as *high-resolution imaging*. There are trade-offs when attempting to achieve high-resolution images, so the operator must have a clear understanding of the effects that scan parameter selections will have on the final image.

Spatial resolution is controlled by scan parameters that directly affect the voxel size. A voxel is a three-dimensional object that is determined when the operator selects the field of view, matrix, and slice thickness. Many voxels are contained within a slice. During Fourier transformation, the components of all signals within a voxel are averaged together to create one signal intensity. The resulting component will be used to convert the data to a two-dimensional pixel for display on conventional CRT screens. The MR operator must choose the voxel volume, through specific selections of matrix and FOV or pixel size, and slice thickness which will yield the least number of signal variations.

The relationship between FOV, matrix, and pixel size can be represented in the following manner:

$$FOV = matrix \times pixel \qquad (4.3)$$

This equation merely states that a change in either FOV, matrix, or pixel size in either the X or the Y dimension of the matrix will have an effect on the other two factors in the equation. Each parameter that contributes to spatial resolution will now be discussed in detail.

Pixel Size

Pixel size, also known as *resolution,* is the two-dimensional version of a voxel. The single most effective method for achieving high-resolution scans is to choose the smallest pixel size appropriate for the anatomy of interest. However, because of the relationship between FOV, matrix, and pixel size, if no other factor in the formula is changed, the FOV can become very small—in fact, too small to accommodate the region of interest, resulting in an aliasing artifact (refer to Chap. 6 for a complete discussion of the aliasing artifact).

On some MRI systems, the operator can select the pixel size independent of the matrix and FOV. In most cases, however, pixel size is calculated from the FOV and matrix chosen, using Eq. (4.3). It is imperative that the operator be familiar with the approximate size of the anatomy being imaged and the differential diagnosis for the clinical situation being presented so that the most appropriate pixel size can be chosen. A general rule of thumb is that the smallest pixel size should be used when imaging small anatomic regions, such as for vascular imaging, extremity imaging, imaging of cranial nerves, or imaging of relatively small pathologic processes.

Table 4-1 shows how pixel size can be altered to improve spatial resolution.

Slice Thickness

In conventional 2DFT imaging, selective slice excitation is a function of creating a gradient magnetic field and apply-

TABLE 4-1 INDIRECT MANIPULATION OF PIXEL SIZE

Matrix	FOV	Result on Pixel Size	Trade-off
Increase PE steps	No change	Decrease in one dimension	Increase scan time Decrease SNR/voxel
Increase RO steps	No change	Decrease in one dimension	Possible decrease in maximum number of slices and/or minimum TE allowed Decrease SNR/voxel
Increase PE and RO steps	No change	Overall decrease	Increase scan time Decrease SNR/voxel
No change	Decrease	Decrease	Decrease SNR/voxel Possible aliasing

ing to the patient an RF pulse specific to each variation of the gradient magnetic field. The position of the slice is frequency-dependent, and the thickness of the slice is determined by the bandwidth (range of frequencies) or the strength of the gradient field. Slice thickness is the third dimension of the voxel, so that variation of the slice thickness contributes to voxel volume.

Enlarging the slice thickness has the effect of reducing spatial resolution, since more tissue elements contained in the slice contribute to the composite signal intensity. This is commonly referred to as the *partial volume effect* and is related to small signals within a larger voxel being obscured by signals from adjacent tissues. Spatial resolution can be optimized by choosing a minimum slice thickness for the area to be imaged. This results in less partial volume averaging and improved tissue conspicuity. However, SNR is reduced, as there are fewer spins contributing to the signal within the smaller slice.

When 3DFT imaging is performed, the slice component of the image is created by another phase-encoding process. This results in resolution of 3D images that can be on the order of one millimeter or less.[1] The advantage of using a 3DFT technique is high-resolution images with sufficient signal. For a more in-depth discussion on 3DFT imaging, the reader is directed to Kramer et al.[1]

Voxel

The voxel is essentially the combination of a pixel with a slice thickness, which creates a volume. The size of the voxel is controlled by the pixel dimensions and the slice thickness, so that a change in any of the three dimensions will have an effect on the volume. While modification of the voxel size results in an alteration in spatial resolution,

a concomitant change in SNR and the amount of partial volume exhibited in the image will also be visible.

Voxels can be equal on all three sides (isotropic) or unequal (anisotropic). The proportions of the voxel can be manipulated to obtain high-resolution scans while maintaining a sufficient amount of signal. For example, if the pixel dimensions are decreased by one-half but the slice thickness is maintained, the voxel becomes rectangular. This has the effect of improving spatial resolution by a factor of 4. If only one side of the voxel was decreased by one-half, spatial resolution would be improved by a factor of 2. If all three dimensions are decreased by one-half, resolution improves by a factor of 8 (see Fig. 4-5). As we will see in Chap. 5, any change in the factors that control spatial resolution has a distinct effect on SNR. In fact, in most cases there is an inverse relationship, so that an increase in spatial resolution will result in a decrease in SNR.

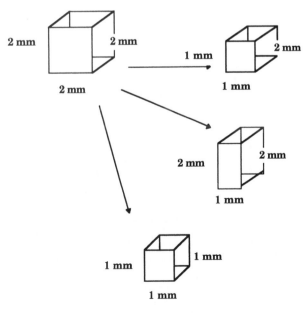

Figure 4-5 Voxel size.

Matrix

The matrix is made up of a great number of individual voxels in the length (PE or Y direction) and width (RO or X direction) of the imaged area. The operator can modify it by selecting the number of phase-encoding steps and the number of data sample points required to yield a desired spatial resolution. The matrix has an effect on the size of the pixel for a given FOV based on the relationship between FOV, matrix, and pixel size given in Eq. (4.3). We know that to obtain high-resolution images, the voxel volume must be as small as possible. In order to accomplish this, the operator must select either small pixel dimensions or minimal slice thickness. However, the operator can also manipulate the matrix or the FOV to obtain high-resolution images. This is an indirect method of choosing the pixel size.

For a given FOV, the matrix can be adjusted so that the number of phase-encoding and/or frequency-encoding steps will yield high-resolution scans. This can be seen in Fig. 4-6.

As can be seen, if the number of phase-encoding and frequency-encoding steps is increased, the pixel size (or voxel volume when the slice thickness dimension is added) decreases, which improves the spatial resolution. The anatomy of interest is essentially diced into more discrete objects, each being assigned a unique gray-scale value. Improving spatial resolution improves contrast resolution, allowing better tissue differentiation. A disadvantage of increasing the matrix for a given FOV is a loss of signal per voxel which may give the image an overall noisy appearance.

The matrix can be adjusted in one or both directions. An alteration in the number of phase-encoding steps will affect scan time, while a change in the readout or frequency direction may affect the maximum number of slices as well as the minimum possible TE for the sequence being performed.

Another benefit of increasing the matrix is a reduction in potential truncation artifacts, which, when present, diminish spatial resolution. Truncation artifacts can occur when there are discontinuous signal intensities, such as interfaces between tissues that have a high versus a low signal. When a lowered matrix is used, the difference between one phase-encoding step (line of data) and another can be quite large, and the information gets "truncated" or cut off during Fourier transform. This produces repetitious dark/white lines that follow the contour of the anatomy. Using the maximum number of PE and RO steps given patient tolerance for the scan time needed will significantly reduce the visibility of this artifact.

Field of View

Field of view (FOV) is an operator-selectable scan parameter which defines the anatomic region of interest. It is selected to cover a particular tissue volume. FOV has an effect on spatial resolution through its dependence on matrix and pixel size, as given by Eq. (4.3). It can be altered in the phase- or frequency-encoding direction or both.

Spatial resolution can be improved by decreasing the FOV for a given matrix selection. If the same number of

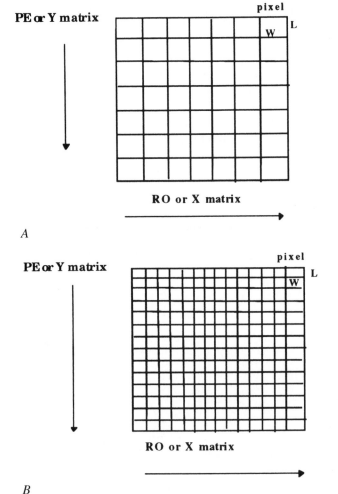

Figure 4-6 Matrix (A) and matrix ×2 (B).

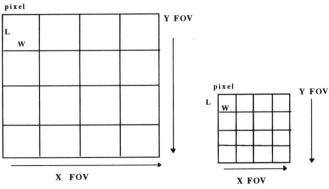

Figure 4-7 FOV.

phase-encoding and frequency-encoding steps are contained in a smaller region of interest, the size of the voxel or pixel is reduced, allowing contrast resolution to be more specific. Figure 4-7 demonstrates this change.

Changes in FOV must be chosen with care, as any decrease in dimensions can adversely affect image quality by introducing wraparound artifacts. Wraparound or aliasing artifacts occur when the FOV is smaller than the area being imaged. The receiver coil still detects signal and incorporates it into the final image.

Improving the spatial resolution of the MR image allows more precise representation of tissue elements. Spatial resolution is controlled by pixel size, slice thickness, matrix selection, and FOV, which are selected by the operator. Knowledge of the size of the anatomic region and the pathologic possibilities is essential in determining the dimensions of the area to be imaged. Table 4-2 is a summary of the effects that specific changes have on spatial resolution. It assumes that no other action has been taken.

Reference

1. Kramer DM, Sweitzer MC: Standard MR pulse sequences: A closer look, in Woodward P, Freimarck R (eds): *MRI for Technologists.* New York: McGraw-Hill, 1995.

Suggested Readings

Elster AD: *Questions and Answers in Magnetic Resonance Imaging.* St. Louis: Mosby, 1994.

Stark DD, Bradley WG Jr: *Magnetic Resonance Imaging.* St. Louis: Mosby, 1988.

Woodward P: Assessing the interaction of image sequence parameters, in Woodward P, Freimarck R (eds): *MRI for Technologists.* New York: McGraw-Hill, 1995.

TABLE 4-2 IMAGE PARAMETER EFFECT OF SPATIAL RESOLUTION

Scan Parameter	Action	Effect on Spatial Resolution
Pixel size	Decrease	Increase
Slice thickness	Decrease	Increase; decrease partial volume averaging
Matrix	Increase	Increase; decrease truncation artifact
FOV	Decrease	Increase

5

Signal-to-Noise Ratio

The *signal-to-noise ratio* (SNR) demands much attention in the MRI business. It is a term that is used to describe the relative contributions of the true signal and of random superimposed signals that we call "noise." When the true signal becomes relatively stronger than noise, the SNR is improved and better images are obtained. Too high an SNR does not necessarily benefit the image. But it can be used to trade for higher-resolution images, shorter scan times, or reduced partial volume effects and truncation artifacts.

The SNR can be improved by either increasing the signal strength or decreasing the noise level. However, signal increases approximately in a linear fashion, whereas noise is random, so in reality, the two are difficult to separate.

Signal is related to the field strength of the operating system and generated by activity associated with energy exchange at the atomic level, typically while imaging the hydrogen nucleus. An increase in field strength by a factor of 2 would theoretically double the SNR, all other factors being equal. Proton density is relatively uniform in soft tissue at a given temperature, so that the only other factor affecting SNR in tissues is the number of nuclei per voxel. Therefore, increasing the size of the voxel can augment signal strength.

Noise is signal that is superimposed on the image (signal that we do not want). It can cause the mean pixel values determined by the true signal to fluctuate, so that some pixels may have a brighter or darker appearance than the mean value would indicate. This suggests that on the image, sufficient noise can smear the edges of tissue interfaces. Small differences in signal intensity that might be important may become impossible to see.

There are two types of noise. The one that we can, to some extent, correct for is the noise which results from variations in the signal created by substances in the body. It is caused by thermal motion in the electrically conductive tissues, causing resistance, which in turn results in a background RF signal. In clinical practice, tissues are the dominant source of noise.

The second type of noise is generated by the system. This is noise which we cannot correct for with our imaging parameters, such as resistance associated with the receiver coil.

There are many factors that contribute to SNR. Many are operator-selectable; some cannot be chosen but are inherent. Those that cannot be selected by the operator include magnetic field strength, magnetic field homogeneity, and proton density.

Magnetic field homogeneity is the product of the field strength of the system times the measured field homogeneity over a clinically useful imaging volume. It is determined during the manufacture of the magnet, which includes the shim process, and also during magnet installation, where additional shimming is required to account for environmental influences. Standards for field homogeneity are specified by both the magnet manufacturer and the MRI vendor. The bottom line is that better absolute field homogeneity results in optimum signal. Interference of the field homogeneity from sources that are magnetically susceptible, such as ferromagnetic objects, can cause fluctuations that result in artifacts and image degradation.

Proton density is relatively uniform within soft tissues. We cannot augment this density by adding more nuclei to tissues. What we can do is to increase the size of the voxel, so that more nuclei are contained in the voxel to produce more signal.

Operator-selectable scan parameters that affect SNR also affect spatial resolution, contrast, and scan time. Trade-offs exist, so that the selection of scan parameters to optimize image quality becomes a balancing act. A discussion of the scan parameters and their effect on SNR follows.

Voxel Volume

As we know from Chapter 4, the voxel is a volume whose dimensions are determined by pixel size and slice thickness. Altering any of the three dimensions will change the size of the voxel. Decreasing its size will result in better spatial resolution, but the SNR will diminish because there will be fewer nuclei contained in the voxel to contribute to the signal. An increase in the voxel size will result in higher SNR but reduced contrast differentiation and lowered spatial resolution. Higher SNR can be achieved by increasing the pixel size, the slice thickness, or both. It can also be achieved indirectly by increasing the FOV or decreasing the matrix, all other factors remaining unchanged. The SNR per voxel has a linear dependence on the volume of the voxel (assuming that one is merely increasing the amount of the same material in the voxel). This means that if we image the same region and double the pixel size, the SNR increases by a factor of 4, or 2×2 (see Fig. 4-5). If we only double the slice thickness, the SNR increases by a factor of 2. In either case, spatial resolution has decreased.

Often, when attempting to increase SNR, spatial resolution can be optimized by altering only one or two dimensions of the voxel, creating an anisotropic voxel. Two important consequences of anisotropic imaging must be considered. The first is related to voxel, matrix, or FOV selections: Rectangular imaging must be oriented to correspond with the anatomy so that no aliasing occurs. The second consequence is related to performing reformatted reconstruction as a postprocess method. The best overall result is obtained when *approximate* cubic voxels are used. This is exemplified when 3DFT imaging techniques are employed, as data sets are all Fourier encoded, resulting in preservation of the original resolution. In 2DFT imaging, where larger slice thicknesses than in 3DFT imaging are generally used, resolution may not be enhanced, resulting in reformatted images without clarity. The important factor is that resolution of the original data be optimum so that reformatted images have image quality that is well defined.

Pulse Sequence Type

The pulse sequence type selected has an effect on SNR because of its association with scan parameter selection. Repetition time (TR), echo time (TE), inversion time (TI), and flip angle (FA) selections are critical in protocol design. Each factor has a unique relationship to the pulse sequence type selected and the ability to produce images with the desired contrast and signal in the least amount of scan time. When an improvement in overall SNR is preferred, any of these factors can be manipulated to achieve this at the expense of contrast or scan time.

There is a common MRI axiom that identifies the relationship between TR, TE, and signal; it defines the signal intensity of a spin echo technique as it relates to nuclear hydrogen proton density $N(H)$ and is seen below:

$$\text{Signal} \propto N(H)\,[1 - \exp(-TR/T1)]\,[\exp(-TE/T2)]$$

where

$N(H)$	Hydrogen proton density values are not field-strength dependent, nor are they consistent between data sets or studies.
$[1 - \exp(-TR/T1)]$	This portion of the equation identifies how TR relates to T1 relaxation times. It is an exponential change in the ratio of TR to T1.
$[\exp(-TE/T2)]$	This is an exponential change in the ratio of TE to T2. It is an inverse of the TR/T1 relationship.

Table 5-1 charts the relationships between TR and T1 and between TE and T2 when the parameters are altered on a typical SE pulse sequence.

TABLE 5-1

Parameter Action	T1 Time	T2 Time	Signal Intensity
TR short	Long		Small
TR short	Short		Moderate
TR long	Short		Large
TR long	Long		Moderate
TE long		Short	Small
TE short		Long	Large
TE long		Long	Moderate
TE short		Short	Moderate

Inversion recovery (IR) techniques use an inverting pulse of 180° to begin the pulse sequence event. Since maximal signal detection is at 90° to the longitudinal plane, the vector must eventually be flipped to the transverse plane for data collection. The interval between the 180° and 90° RF pulses is the contrast controlling parameter in these types of sequences (refer to Chap. 3 for more detail regarding contrast control). As can be seen in Fig. 5-1, image signal intensity can be manipulated by changing the TI time.

Since the hydrogen protons in fat contribute to significant signal, using a TI time that is approximately at the null point of fat will produce images that are fairly signal-starved. If clinical indication dictates fat-suppression techniques to enhance pathology, a STIR (short-TI inversion recovery) sequence satisfies the objective, even though the signal may be lacking.

Gradient echo or field echo imaging is commonly performed using flip angles that are less than 90°. Since there are fewer spins contributing to the signal when a shorter flip angle is used, images with less SNR are generated. Signal can be improved when using GRE sequences with short flip angles by maximizing voxel volume. This can be accomplished in the usual method by increasing the dimensions of the voxel or by performing 3DFT imaging techniques. Since the purpose of this technique is to obtain images with sufficient SNR by selective excitation of one large slice that is then phase-encoded to create multiple thin slices, spatial resolution can be maintained without compromising SNR. Another method that is becoming popular is to increase the slice thickness for acquisition purposes, then use a reconstruction process that produces additional thin slices from the original information.

TABLE 5-2

Number of Acquisitions	SNR Factor	Improvement, Percent
1	Standard of 1.00	—
2	1.41	41
3	1.73	73
4	2.0	100
5	2.24	124
6	2.45	145
7	2.65	165
8	2.83	183

Number of Averages (N_{acq} or NA)

A method commonly used to improve SNR is to increase the total number of planar acquisitions of N_{acq} per phase-encode step. Essentially, the data collection process is repeated without changing the phase-encode gradient strength. Signal will add linearly, while statistical noise, which is random, adds incoherently, so that SNR improves only by the square root of the factor by which the N_{acq} was changed ($SNR \propto \sqrt{N_{acq}}$). Stated differently, this means that if one doubles the number of acquisitions, signal improves by only $\sqrt{2}$, or 41 percent. We know that the N_{acq} is used to calculate total scan time, so that scan time also doubles in this example. To improve SNR by 100 percent, one must use at least $4N_{acq}$; however, critical scan-time factors must be acknowledged with respect to patient tolerance. Fast scan techniques (Chap. 7) allow significant increases in the number of planar acquisitions without compromising scan time. Table 5-2 shows the SNR improvement with increases in N_{acq}.

It may not be effective to increase the N_{acq} beyond a time factor that most patients would find acceptable. Even if the patient is tolerant of the procedure, many physiologic processes continue that will contribute to noise and for which we cannot completely compensate.

Number of Phase-Encoding Steps (PE)

The selection of the number of phase-encoding steps is primarily dependent on the spatial resolution desired in

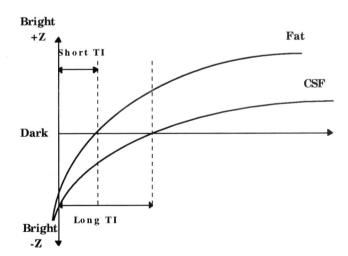

Figure 5-1 Contrast control using short versus long TI.

the Y direction of the matrix. The more PE steps used per FOV selection, the smaller the voxel size, which improves resolution. There are two factors affecting SNR which must be considered when increasing the number of PE steps. One is that an increase in PE steps over the same original FOV will result in a decrease in SNR per voxel volume. The second is that increasing the number of PE steps increases the number of planar data acquisitions (N_{acq}) that contribute to averaging. The potential increase in SNR resulting from this is similar to the increase seen when the number of acquisitions is increased; that is, the increase is proportional to the square root of the change factor ($SNR \propto \sqrt{PE}$). However, since voxel volume must be considered, the overall percent improvement of SNR may not be significant.

Increasing the number of phase-encoding steps also increases scan time, so that patient tolerance for the exam must be considered. In addition, since the phase-encoding gradient results in a slightly different degree of change for each N_{acq}, there is no guarantee that for each data collection the moving spins (blood flow, CSF, respirations, etc.) will be at their original location.

There are many advantages to increasing the number of phase-encoding steps: an overall increase in SNR on the image, improved spatial resolution, and a potential decrease in truncation artifact visibility. An educated selection of this scan parameter will result in optimum image quality.

Number of Data Samples (RO)

The number of data samples (frequency encoding or *readout*), like the number of phase-encoding steps, is selected for the effect it will have on spatial resolution in the X direction of the matrix. It is the point during the timed pulse sequence at which the time-varying signal is sampled. It is performed many times during the collection of signal from the echo. Aside from voxel volume effects, increasing the number of RO steps improves $SNR \propto \sqrt{RO}$ (just like increasing the number of PE steps or N_{acq}) by yielding more information in the form of data samples that will be used to reconstruct an image. The voxel volume effect is related to an increase in the total number of data samples per FOV selection and works similarly to increasing the number of PE steps: The voxel volume decreases, resulting in a decrease in SNR per volume. Unlike when the number of PE steps is increased, there is no time penalty when the number of RO steps is increased,

so that this scan parameter can be manipulated to improve SNR and spatial resolution without affecting the scan time.

Bandwidth

The bandwidth is the range of frequencies included in the acquired data. It is determined in part by the strength of the readout gradient and the data sampling rate (time between successive samples) and is specific to the MR imaging system. It can be calculated using the following equation:

$$\text{Bandwidth} = \frac{\text{Sample rate}}{\text{\#RO samples}}$$

It has no effect on the strength of the signal but is intimately related to noise, so that SNR is affected by bandwidth. Noise is present in all frequencies, so that if the range of frequencies measured is large, more statistical noise will contribute to the signal, resulting in a decrease in the SNR. The bandwidth is inversely proportional to the total sampling time, so that if the bandwidth is halved, the time interval between samples is doubled. This results in an increase in SNR per voxel of $\sqrt{2}$, or a 41 percent higher signal.

There are some disadvantages to using narrow-bandwidth sequences, however. In order to decrease the bandwidth, readout or sampling time is increased. Refocusing and balancing pulses are performed as usual before echo collection with the readout gradient centered on the echo. The amplitude of the readout gradient is reduced in narrow-bandwidth sequences to allow nuclear precessional frequency information to be incorporated in the new lower bandwidth. This requires more time in the pulse sequence, so that the echo time necessarily becomes longer. This may in fact lead to a reduction in slices per TR.

Chemical shift artifact is increased when using narrow-bandwidth sequences, especially at high field strengths, where this phenomenon is more ubiquitous (see Chap. 6 for more detail on chemical shift artifact). Use of a fat-suppression sequence with narrow-bandwidth imaging reduces this artifact.

Increased motion artifact from flow and other physiologic motion has been associated with the use of narrow-bandwidth imaging. However, with the improvement in overall SNR, total scan time can be decreased by lowering the number of acquisitions, which will reduce motion artifacts. Additionally, variable-bandwidth selections that allow the second echo to incorporate narrow-bandwidth techniques will result in improvement of the signal in the echo.

Narrow-bandwidth imaging has improved MRI technology by limiting noise in the sampled data. It comes in a variety of forms, so that referral to the operator's guide for the MRI system in use is imperative.

The signal-to-noise ratio is an important image quality criterion for many MRI investigators. It can be used to produce beautiful images with little contrast or can be traded for images with shorter scan times, higher resolution, and fewer artifacts.

Table 5-3 charts the effect scan parameter selections have on SNR, contrast, resolution, artifacts, and scan time.

TABLE 5-3 SCAN PARAMETER SELECTIONS

Scan Parameter	Action	Effect on SNR	Effect on Contrast	Effect on Spatial Resolution	Artifacts	Scan Time
TR	Increase	Increase	Decrease T1; increase T2 effects; increase $N(H)$	No real effect	Increase motion/flow	Increase
TE	Increase	Decrease	Increase T2; decrease T1 effects	No real effect	Increase motion/flow	No change
TI	Increase	Possible increase in fat signal	Increase T1	No real effect	Increase motion/flow	No change unless TR increased
FA	Increase	Increase	Increase T1; decrease T2°	No real effect	No change	No change unless TR increased
ETL	Increase	Decrease due to T2 effects from later echoes	Increase contrast mix	Decrease via increase artifact	Increase blurring	Decrease
ETE	Increase	Decrease	Increase T2	No change	No change	No change
ETS	Increase	Decrease due to T2 effects from later echoes	Increase contrast mix but decrease contrast control	Decrease via increase artifact	Increase blurring	No change
N_{acq}	Increase	Increase by $\sqrt{\ }$	None	Increase	Decrease FID	Increase
PE steps	Increase	Increase by $\sqrt{\ }$; decrease/voxel	Overall increase due to small pixel with more precise gray-scale value	Increase	Decrease truncation	Increase
RO steps	Increase	Increase $\sqrt{\ }$; decrease/voxel	Overall increase due to small pixel with more precise gray-scale value	Increase	Decrease aliasing	No change
FOV	Increase	Increase	Decrease due to larger pixel size with less precision	General decrease	Decrease aliasing	No change
Slice thickness (2DFT)	Increase	Increase	Decrease due to partial volume effect	Decrease via increase artifact, which affects contrast	Increase partial volume effect	No change
Partitions/slab (3DFT)	Increase	Decrease	Increase	Increase due to thinner slices per slab	No change	Increase
Bandwidth	Increase	Increase by $\sqrt{\ }$	May allow increase in TE/T2	Decrease via increase artifact	Increase chemical shift	No change

Suggested Readings

Elster AD: *Questions and Answers in Magnetic Resonance Imaging.* St. Louis: Mosby, 1994.

Hendrick, RE: Signal-to-noise in MRI, March 1990.

Oldendorf W, Oldendorf W Jr: *Basics of Magnetic Resonance Imaging.* Boston: Martinus Nijhoff Publishing, 1988.

Schulz RA: A primer on resolution/field of view/coverage/imaging time in MRI.

Stark DD, Bradley WG Jr.: *Magnetic Resonance Imaging.* St. Louis: Mosby, 1988.

Sweitzer JC, Kramer DM: Standard MR pulse sequences: A closer look, in Woodward P, Freimarck R (eds): *MRI for Technologists.* New York: McGraw-Hill, 1995.

Wehrli FW, MacFall JR, Newton TH: Parameters determining the appearance of NMR images.

Woodward P: Assessing the interaction of image sequence parameters, in Woodward P, Freimarck R (eds): *MRI for Technologists.* New York: McGraw-Hill, 1995.

Young SW: *Magnetic Resonance Imaging Basic Principles,* 2d ed. New York: Raven Press, 1988.

6

Artifacts

The introduction of magnetic resonance in the mid-eighties brought a sophistication to the diagnostic imaging field that has been unsurpassed. To put the technique of MRI in simple terms, radio-frequency energy is directed into the patient, who is in the confines of a strong external magnetic field. This RF energy is altered by stationary tissues, vascular structures, and magnetic fields. It then is returned and collected to create a clinically useful image. However, while the return signal carries an accurate representation of three-dimensional structures in the patient's body, it can also carry false information that can obscure the signal from the tissues. This false information is called an *artifact,* and it sometimes mimics pathology.

There are many different artifacts associated with magnetic resonance imaging that can be prevented if they are understood. It is the responsibility of the operator to be familiar with artifacts so that steps can be used to reduce the effects. This chapter is intended to identify the most common artifacts seen in MR imaging over which there is reasonable operator control. The appearance and origin of each artifact will be discussed, along with any compensatory measures that can be taken to minimize or eliminate the artifact. Refer to Chap. 12 for a thorough description of artifact-suppression techniques.

Motion

The most common artifact seen in MRI is caused by motion, which is most often the result of physiologic processes such as respiration and flow dynamics or of patient movement. In the phase-encoding direction, motion produces ghosting of the body part in which the motion occurred. It appears as if the anatomy has reproduced itself many times in the phase-encoding direction (see Fig. 6-1). Motion can also cause blurring in the direction of motion that is proportional to the distance moved. This may result in loss of detail as a result of the general fuzziness of the image.

MR images are sensitive to motion because they are acquired during a time sequence. Motion can occur during or between RF pulses, during data sampling, or between phase-encode steps. Since movement of spins occurs over time (for example, heart rate ∼ 72 beats/60 s; respirations ∼ 14/60 s) and the images are collected during a timed sequence, the spins at the beginning of the acquisition are never at the same position at the end of the acquisition. When the data are collected, they contain information with regard to the phase, frequency, and amplitude of the signal. This is based on the original position of the spins in the phase direction; however, since phase information is collected a multitude of times at distinct intervals, there is a phase shift that will cause the spins' signal to be mismapped in the phase-encode direction. Essentially, the spins that originally absorbed RF energy at the beginning of the pulse sequence are no longer available to reemit the energy, and a flow artifact is generated.

These ghost images are a result of a failure of gradients to completely eliminate the phase contribution of either the slice select or frequency-encoding gradients when motion occurs in these planes. Motion can originate from fast flow (i.e., arterial), pulsatile flow (cerebral spinal fluid), slow flow (i.e., venous and lymphatic), cardiac

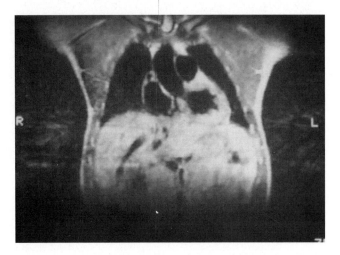

Figure 6-1 Coronal body shows generalized motion in the phase-encoding direction, right to left.

movement, respirations, peristalsis, and the uncooperative patient (see Fig. 6-2).

Motion artifact can also appear as a result of gradient coil instability. Gradient coils are housed in a separate facade of the MR system. In superconductive magnet systems, they reside in a cylindrical compartment that is within the magnet coil housing. An enormous amount of vibration is generated during the NMR experiment as a result of the interaction of the gradient coils with the external magnet field. If the gradient coil housing is not secure, motion artifact can present that looks very similar to patient motion. However, a clue to its origin is that the motion occurs regardless of patient tolerance or sequence, and the image does not appear to have a generalized appearance of patient motion.

Solutions

Presaturation techniques which saturate flowing spins with RF so that they cannot contribute signal may be used to minimize or eliminate flow artifact. They can be directed perpendicular to the slice or in the same direction as the slice. This technique is valuable for reducing the

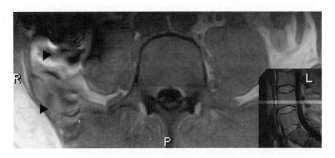

Figure 6-2 Motion artifact from peristalsis and the inferior vena cava is portrayed at edge of arrows, on right.

contribution of respiration and peristalsis in abdominal imaging as well as motion artifacts from moving spins such as blood flow.

Gradient moment nulling or *flow compensation* may be used to compensate for spin phase shifts which accumulate while under the influence of a gradient. A balanced reversal of the effect of the normal gradients is introduced, so that a phase shift does not occur. This technique is useful when CSF pulsatile flow or venous flow is the primary source of the artifact.

Artifacts produced by cardiac motion can be minimized with *ECG triggering*, which is used to synchronize data collection with the heart rate. Essentially, data acquisition occurs only during the time in which minimal hemodynamic effects occur.

The proper choice of parameters (i.e., *breath-hold imaging* and *short TR/TE sequences*) helps eliminate the possibility of motion artifact due to short scanning times. Narrow-bandwidth or hybrid echo sequences help decrease motion artifacts by decreasing scan time (narrow-bandwidth technology may allow a reduction in the number of acquisitions). Glucagon administration to minimize peristalsis in the bowel has been advocated by some clinicians.

Fast scanning techniques will greatly affect the ability to produce T2-weighted sequences in the shortest possible scan times. Respiration and peristalsis become more manageable, thereby increasing the success of abdominal imaging. A complete description of fast scan techniques can be found in Chap. 7.

A *decrease in the number of acquisitions* will decrease scan time, which will decrease the amount of time the spins are allowed to accumulate a phase shift. This reduces motion artifacts, but will limit the amount of noise averaged out of the resultant image.

Reorientation of the phase- versus frequency-encoding gradient can help to minimize motion artifact that is not occurring in the phase-encode direction. For example, when imaging for a sagittal lumbar spine, motion can be a result of respirations, peristalsis, CSF pulsations, or arterial/venous flow. When the phase-encoding gradient is directed superior/inferior, motion from breathing, peristalsis, and the heart can be minimized. Flow artifact occurring in the superior-to-inferior direction may still be present, but it will not be a significant source of image degradation.

Sponges and other support devices can significantly reduce patient motion. By making the patient comfortable before initiation of the scan and by effectively blocking routes of movement, potential patient motion can be hindered.

Sedation can be used by qualified personnel to minimize patient motion. It is important to monitor the patient during a sedative-induced procedure and be prepared for unexpected medical complications.

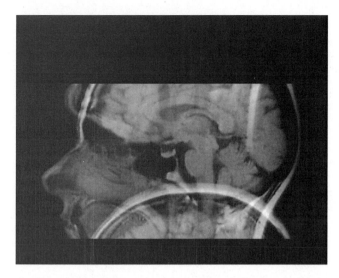

Figure 6-3 An FOV of 13 cm is used in the superior-to-inferior direction of the head, inadequately covering the anatomic region and causing aliasing.

Aliasing

Aliasing, also called *wraparound artifact*, occurs when the diameter of the object exceeds the field of view (see Fig. 6-3).

When imaging, there is a finite number of frequencies used to sample the data. These data will have phase, frequency, and amplitude information that will be used to determine where in the matrix the signal will be assigned. The matrix size determines the number of assigned slots available. Aliasing is a result of uncertainty in the assignment of the samples to these slots.

This is a result of the fact that data from high-frequency signals can have the same amplitude as data from low-frequency signals, and so the Fourier transform is unable to differentiate the two. If anatomy being imaged is outside the selected field of view, but within the range of the imaging coil, the region outside will be assigned an ambiguous sample slot, resulting in at least two frequencies being equal. Their assigned locations within the matrix will be superimposed, and the region which extended outside the field of view will now appear in the image, but on the opposite side.

Solution

Increasing the field of view allows the entire region of interest to be sampled appropriately, so that no aliasing occurs. Since more sample slots are available, there is less possibility for two frequencies to have the same values and therefore the same spatial location.

Aliasing generally occurs in the phase-encoding direction, where there are no associated frequency filters. Most MR systems use frequency filters in the frequency-encoding direction to filter data that are external to the field of view and outside a particular frequency range. In addition, since there is no time penalty associated with an increase in the readout steps (matrix in the X direction), oversampling in the frequency-encoding direction is commonly performed to help eliminate aliasing in that direction. A *change in phase-encoding and frequency-encoding axes* relative to the patient size can better accommodate the area of interest if chosen with care by taking advantage of oversampling and frequency filters.

Surface coils can minimize aliasing artifacts because the coil does not receive signal beyond its radius. By selecting a coil size that fits the image region and by positioning that region in the center of the coil, potential aliasing artifacts can be eliminated.

The use of *antialiasing techniques* such as no-phase wrap and oversampling in the frequency-encoding direction can greatly reduce wraparound artifact. These techniques use increased data sample levels during acquisition. Since the original field of view is much smaller than the acquired region, only the data samples within the FOV are used to create the image. Information obtained outside the region of interest has been given distinct spatial locations and can be easily separated from the data of interest. In this way, no aliasing is allowed. While antialiasing techniques are very effective, the increase in the number of phase-encoding steps used in the no-phase wrap technique results in an increase in scan time. This can be offset by using fewer total acquisitions (reduce N_{acq}). Since doubling the number of phase-encoding steps or the number of acquisitions results in an improvement in SNR of 41 percent, halving the N_{acq} when using no-phase wrap techniques keeps scan time at a minimum without adversely affecting the SNR (see Chap. 5). Oversampling in the frequency-encoding direction does not pose any time penalty and is often automatically incorporated into pulse sequences.

Metal

Metals have the ability to produce significant artifacts that are among the most common artifacts seen in MRI. Some metals that are placed in the magnet distort the static magnetic field because of their own intrinsic magnetic

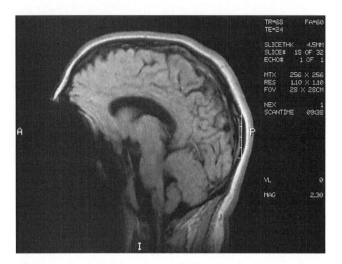

Figure 6-4 Metallic artifact caused by ferromagnetic substance.

properties. Metals that do not have these properties (that is, nonmagnetic metals) may also distort the static field because of inherent inductive properties that are initiated by the gradient fields.

Metals are classified as ferromagnetic, paramagnetic, and diamagnetic. Ferromagnetic metals have the ability to interact with the static magnetic field enough to highly concentrate field flux lines (see Fig. 6-4). Examples of ferromagnetics are iron, cobalt, and nickel. Substances that contain only 11 percent nickel are considered ferromagnetic.

Paramagnetic metals concentrate magnetic lines of force to a lesser extent than do ferromagnetics. Injectable forms of paramagnetics are gadolinium and manganese. Noninjectable paramagnetics include titanium, platinum, and iridium. These materials will not distort the static magnetic field to the extent that ferromagnetics will, but they will have an effect on the uniformity of the field that is sufficient to cause artifacts.

Diamagnetic materials, such as gold, zinc, mercury, and copper, can alter the static field homogeneity, but significantly less than ferromagnetic or paramagnetic substances. While they are generally considered to pose little problem with respect to artifact production, a large amount of diamagnetic material can produce the same effect as a microscopic amount of iron. This is exemplified by the artifacts produced by mascara or eyeliner, which can be dramatic.[1] Diamagnetic changes also occur in the body at edge interfaces where signal intensities are sufficiently different, such as between air and tissue, bone and tissue, and liquid and tissue. These regions of the body include the areas near the pituitary, sinuses, lungs, bowel, and bone. A term that is used to describe this phenomenon is *magnetic susceptibility*. It describes the intensity of the induced magnetization in an object exposed to an external magnetic field.

Because of their conductive nature, diamagnetics' ability to absorb and reemit RF energy is also a concern, and this should be considered a safety issue. For example, a gold chain that is not removed for an MR examination can cause physical burns to a patient in locations where it is in contact with skin as a result of the conductive property of gold.

Materials that do not inherently exhibit magnetic properties may still cause artifacts that have the appearance of metallic artifacts. Based on the concept of electromagnetism, gradient magnetic fields can induce electric currents in the nonmagnetic substance, creating a local magnetic field. This field can cause distortion of the static magnetic field, which in turn causes misregistration in the spatial location of the data (see Fig. 6-5).

Any metal that is known to be attracted to the static magnetic field while outside of the magnet has the potential for causing metallic artifacts when within the magnet's field of view. Even if no artifact is generated, the signal-to-noise ratio can be reduced significantly. For this reason, it is recommended that the patient be issued MR-compatible clothing (clothing that does not contain metallic components that could interfere with the production of optimal image quality). Furthermore, the patient should not have on the body any substance such as shaving gel, self-tanning lotion, or cosmetics such as eye shadows or eyeliners that contain iron oxide materials, since these materials have been shown to generate metallic artifacts in some cases. Of greater importance is the potential for any metal-containing object to cause injury or discomfort to patients or personnel. The MR operator is encouraged to read *Magnetic Resonance Imaging Bioeffects,*

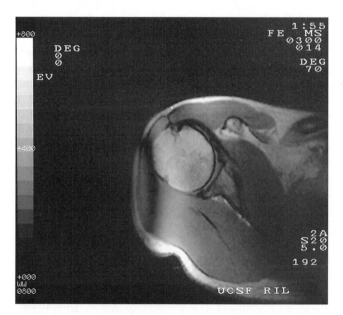

Figure 6-5 Magnetic susceptibility artifact caused by shoulder coil.

**TABLE 6-1 OBJECTS THAT CAN PRODUCE
METALLIC ARTIFACTS**

Pulse oximeter	Pager	ID badge	Nail clipper
Shrapnel	Hearing aid	Calculator	Key
Knife	Jewelry	Hairpin	Paper money
Cigarette lighter	Scissors	Prosthesis	Coins
Stethoscope	Pens/pencils	Watch	Brassiere
Steel shoe tips/heels	Zippers	Eyeliner	Self-tanning lotion

Safety, and Patient Management, by Frank Shellock, Ph.D., and Emanuel Kanal, M.D., published by Raven Press.

Table 6-1 is a partial list of objects that have been reported to be attracted to the magnetic field and that can produce artifacts.

Artifacts produced by metals manifest themselves in a number of ways within the same image. A signal void where the metal is located is seen, with a high-intensity signal adjacent to the void, where the signal has been misregistered (see Fig. 6-6). This combination, in turn, produces a truncation artifact (a complete description of the truncation artifact is given later in this chapter). Distortion and overall signal degradation are also noted.

In addition, local magnetic field distortions can also cause rapid T2 dephasing, which causes increased loss of signal. If the original field homogeneity is good, image quality suffers less from the effects of T2 dephasing. Many pulse sequences, such as sequences that use gradient echoes to focus the spins, are highly susceptible to changes in field homogeneity (see Fig. 6-7).

Solutions

Screening the patient adequately for metal helps to eliminate the possibility of introducing objects that may have an effect on the magnetic field into the scan room. Jewelry, hair devices, surgical implants, dentures, and even

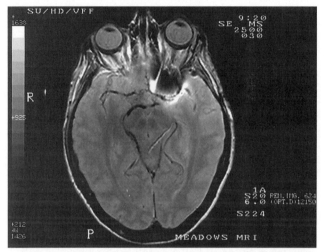

A

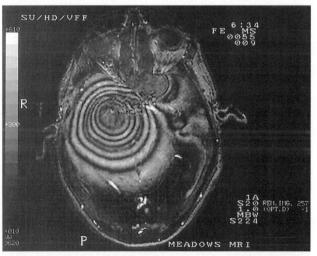

B

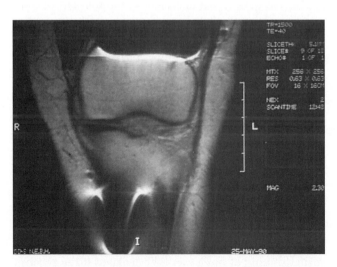

Figure 6-6 Image shows area of signal void, in which the metal is located, a high-intensity signal caused by signal misregistration, truncation artifact caused by signal discontinuity, and image distortion.

Figure 6-7 *A.* Patient denied metallic foreign body; however, the conventional SE image shows a metallic artifact. *B.* A gradient echo sequence on the same patient shows significantly more artifact.

some clothing can cause warping of the static magnetic field as a result of their magnetic properties. Patients should be issued clothing that has been determined to be free of any substance that may have an effect on the magnetic field and should remove any item that may cause distortion of the static magnetic field.

If scanning a patient with a metallic object is unavoidable, and no harm to the patient will result, protocol determination should be based on *pulse sequences* that are not extremely susceptible to inhomogeneities in the magnetic field such as conventional spin echo techniques. Sequences such as gradient echo techniques and narrow-bandwidth technology tend to exaggerate the metallic artifact. In fact, gradient echo imaging is used by some clinicians to *help* the diagnostic process when looking for acute or chronic hemorrhage. Since blood in its acute stage or when hemosiderin is present is highly ferromagnetic, using a gradient echo sequence can produce an artifact that has the appearance of metal that has been introduced into the magnetic field, making the blood more conspicuous.

Chemical Shift

Chemical shift artifact appears as asymmetric dark and light bands along the frequency axis of fat/water interfaces (see Fig. 6-8). It is most often associated with a difference in the Larmor frequency of the hydrogen molecules in fat and water that occur within the same pixel. It can also manifest at interfaces between substances whose chemical shift is significantly different, such as water–Pantopaque and water–silicone interfaces. This difference in precessional frequency is due to the location of the electron or-

bit of the atom relative to the nucleus. When the electron orbit is close to the nucleus, as in lipids, there is a stronger magnetic shielding effect on the nucleus by the electron, which in turn reduces the magnetic susceptibility of the nucleus to the imaging process, thus lowering the precessional frequency of fat. The hydrogen atom attached to oxygen in the water molecule has electron clouds that are further away from the nucleus, resulting in less shielding of the nucleus from the effects of the applied magnetic field, which in turn will be strong. The precessional frequency of the nucleus in water will be higher.

There is a 3.5-ppm chemical shift between the resonant frequency of the hydrogen protons in fat and in water, which will depend on the applied magnetic field. The higher the magnetic field, the greater the frequency, resulting in a significant shift of the fat/water interface by several pixels from the original spatial location. Chemical shift can be calculated using the following equation:

$$\Delta f = \text{operating frequency in MHz} \times 3.5 \text{ ppm}$$

Examples:

0.5 T: $\Delta f = (21 \text{ MHz}) (3.5 \text{ ppm})$
$= (21 \times 10^6 \text{ Hz}) (3.5 \times 10^{-6}) = 74 \text{ Hz}$

1.5 T: $\Delta f = (64 \text{ MHz}) (3.5 \text{ ppm})$
$= (64 \times 10^6 \text{ Hz}) (3.5 \text{ } 10^{-6}) = 224 \text{ Hz}$

The chemical shift at a magnetic field of 0.5 T with an operating frequency of 21 MHz will be about 74 Hz, whereas at a field strength of 1.5 T, the chemical shift is about 224 Hz.

The difference in the two frequencies is small, and excitation of both proton fractions occurs at the excitation radio frequency used for slice selection. When the frequency gradient is applied, the molecules in the selected slice increase or decrease their frequency of precession pending their position linearly. Since the hydrogen molecule in fat is already precessing more slowly for its location following the application of the gradient, the signal from fat will be assumed to originate from an incorrect location: It will appear to have arisen from water protons in another voxel that is residing at the lower part of the gradient field. The artifact will be seen as a band that is white or dark and is one to several pixels in width. It is seen at edge interfaces of water and fat, such as around the kidneys, at optic nerves, and at the disk versus vertebral body edge in the frequency-encoding direction. The loss of edge symmetry results in a perceived loss of spatial resolution as well.

Chemical shift causes a spatial shifting that is sensitive to the static magnetic field strength. The amount of spatial shifting of pixels can be calculated if the receiver bandwidth, the number of data samples (matrix in the frequency-encoding direction), and the chemical shift between the substances at a particular field strength are known. For example, if an image with 256 frequency-en-

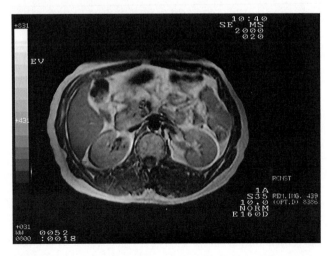

Figure 6-8 Chemical shift artifact seen at right edge of liver and kidney, in the readout direction (small arrowheads).

coding steps was sampled using 32 kHz, the bandwidth per pixel would be 32,000/256, or 125 Hz. The pixel shift at 1.5 T can be calculated as 224 Hz/125 Hz, or 1.8 pixels. At 0.5 T, the same calculation would yield a 0.6-pixel shift. If the receiver bandwidth is reduced by half, the pixel shift approximately doubles.

Examples:

1.5 T: Bandwidth calculation

$$\frac{256 \text{ RO pixels}}{16,000 \text{ Hz}} = 62.5 \text{ Hz/pixel}$$

Pixel shift calculation

$$\frac{62.5 \text{ Hz}}{224 \text{ Hz}} = 3.5 \text{ pixels}$$

0.5 T: Bandwidth calculation

$$\frac{256 \text{ RO pixels}}{16,000 \text{ Hz}} = 62.5 \text{ Hz/pixel}$$

Pixel shift calculation

$$\frac{62.5 \text{ Hz}}{74 \text{ Hz}} = 0.6 \text{ pixel}$$

From the equations above, it can be deduced that not only does an increase in the strength of the operating magnetic field have an effect on the chemical shift artifact, but the use of narrow-bandwidth imaging techniques will cause an increase in pixel shift as well. When the combination of high field imaging and narrow-bandwidth technology is used, pixel shift, resulting in the chemical shift artifact, can be significant.

Spatial shifting does occur in the phase-encoding direction as well; however, there is no cumulative phase shift from fat protons relative to water protons in conventional spin echo and gradient echo imaging. The phase difference is constant at a given location between phase-encoding steps. Additionally, the Fourier transform takes the phase difference into account in assigning spatial location to a signal in this direction, so that no fat-water misregistration occurs along the phase-encoding axis.[2]

Solution

Chemical shift artifacts are a common phenomenon in MR imaging, but they are more pronounced at high magnetic fields and with narrow-bandwidth imaging techniques. Familiarity with the appearance of this artifact should obviate major difficulties in image interpretation. If difficulties arise, there are several strategies that are useful in minimizing this artifact.

A change in *scan direction* (phase- versus frequency-encoding direction) can help to minimize chemical shift artifact by placing the scan in a direction that causes the least amount of interference. Care must be taken when using the strategy, as swapping encoding axes may direct flow-related artifacts into the area of interest or may result in aliasing artifacts.

A reduction in the size of the artifact can be accomplished by increasing the total receiver bandwidth. This is sometimes referred to as using a *steeper readout gradient alignment.* It keeps the chemical shift artifacts at a more tolerable level. This method is dependent on the capability of the imaging system to change gradient strengths (variable or selectable bandwidth technology) and to tolerate the additional strain placed on the gradients.

The use of *specialized pulse sequences* can result in complete separation of fat and water or elimination of signal from fat altogether. *STIR* (short-TI inversion recovery) sequences can eliminate chemical shift artifact by suppressing the signal from fat completely. *Dixon or modified Dixon techniques* use spin echo technology to collect only the signal from either fat or water by sampling the data at a unique point in the TR relative to the specific frequency, thus reducing the artifact. *Chemical shift "out-of-phase"* imaging techniques (see Chap. 10) use gradient echo refocusing techniques, in which fat and water protons go in and out of phase with one another as a function of echo time.[3] The echo time used during data sampling is chosen specifically to produce the phase cancellation phenomenon in which fat and water signals subtract from one another, producing a signal void. Out-of-phase gradient echo imaging is not limited to the frequency-encoding direction, so that the "chemical shift artifact" is essentially seen symmetrically at all fat/water interfaces. The images appear as if the edges of these interfaces have been outlined in black.

Truncation Artifact and Gibbs Ringing

Truncation is a term used to describe the aspect of contraction, reduction, or cut. In MRI, it appears as an edge artifact that consists of multiple high- and low-intensity bands that parallel areas of abrupt changes in signal intensity, such as the cortex of bone and the bone marrow. It also produces false widening of the edge interface and distortion of tissues close to the interface.

This artificial widening can mimic pathology in the spinal cord, such as a syrinx or spinal canal narrowing. The amount or duplicity of the artifact is related to the acquisition matrix used by the system, with lower matrices contributing to an increase in the artifact. Even though the artifact is related to the entire acquisition matrix, it is

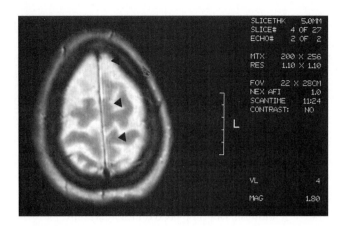

Figure 6-9 Repetitious banding (small arrowheads) seen at interface of brain tissue and falx. Acquisition matrix used 200 phase-encoding steps.

most often seen in the phase-encoding direction, where there is normally less data sampling than in the readout or frequency-encoding direction (see Fig. 6-9).

Truncation artifact is often referred to as *Gibbs ringing;* however, even though both artifacts present similarly, Gibbs ringing is a phenomenon that is inherent to MR data acquisition and cannot be eliminated, whereas the truncation artifact can be eliminated. Gibbs ringing is more conspicuous because higher frequencies that exist at boundaries of low- and high-intensity signals cannot all be sampled. This results in a ringing artifact at that boundary.

The truncation of the Fourier series in MRI when using a reduced number of phase-encoding steps may result in a reconstruction misregistration of the original object. An object with a gradual change in signal intensity, which originates from the sum of sine and cosine waves that have unique frequencies and amplitudes, will be processed more accurately by the Fourier transform. Where there is an abrupt change in signal intensity, such as at the bone cortex and marrow interface, signal is imprecisely represented at the interface and adjacent tissues by oscillating waves that overshoot and undershoot the ideal intensity. The first peak adjacent to the tissue signal discontinuity always overshoots the ideal intensity to a greater degree than subsequent peaks. This is the Gibbs phenomenon, and it will always occur regardless of the matrix chosen.

Solution

Increasing the acquisition matrix results in less signal difference between data sample rows, thus diminishing the intensity of the truncation artifact. This will have no effect on Gibbs ringing, however.

Decreasing pixel size will result in an increase in the ability of the Fourier transform to distinguish differences in signal intensities, since the different objects may have a better chance of residing in individual pixels.

Reconstruction algorithms which modify the phases of the complex data samples can be used to minimize the appearance of truncation artifacts and Gibbs ringing by smoothing edge interfaces. However, if used to minimize truncation artifacts resulting from acquisition with a reduced matrix, this smoothing effect may further degrade image detail by giving the low-resolution image an overall blurred appearance.

Use of *compensatory low-pass filters* can eliminate the truncation artifact by filtering high-frequency signals. They will not filter the first overshoot peak that is the origin of the Gibbs phenomenon, however, and so they will not be effective in Gibbs ringing and may in fact increase the artifact.

Radio-Frequency Artifact

Radio-frequency artifacts can manifest in a number of different ways. They can appear as discrete areas of noise, such as a continuous discrete line through the image perpendicular to the readout direction, or as a general increase in the background noise in either the phase or the readout direction. They often appear as alternating dark and light pixels along one or more frequency-encode lines, mimicking a zipper, and so they are sometimes referred to as *zipper artifacts* (see Fig. 6-10).

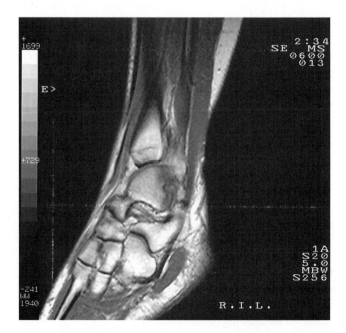

Figure 6-10 Multiple discrete RF artifacts.

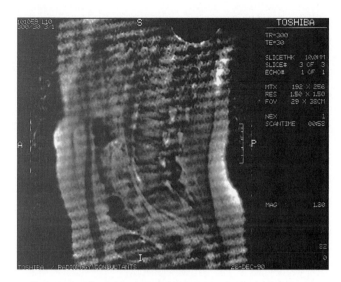

Figure 6-11 Significant RF artifact. Also note the area of metallic artifact at the superior/posterior edge of the image.

When multiple frequencies are affected, overall image quality may suffer in a diffuse manner. In this case, the radio-frequency artifacts may give the appearance of material like corduroy or herringbone. The pattern is a result of reconstruction of the extraneous signals that are then superimposed on the image (see Fig. 6-11).

RF artifacts may result from RF penetration of the scanning environment, interference caused by operation of electronic devices in the scanning environment (e.g., cryogenic meters), interference caused by any material exhibiting properties that produce static electricity (e.g., wool blankets or nylons) (see Fig. 6-12), or interference caused by AC fluctuations (e.g., faulty light bulbs).

Basically, any extraneous RF energy near the operating frequency of the MR imaging system can be detected

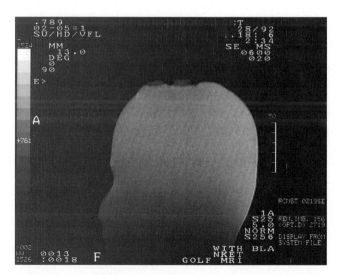

Figure 6-12 Herringbone appearance caused by static electricity from a wool blanket.

and used in producing the final image. In midfield systems, such as 0.5 T, amateur radio transmitters operating between 21.00 and 21.145 MHz can affect resonance. At high field strength (1.5 T), television channels ranging from 60 to 66 MHz can interfere with MRI. The RF lines of interference will be parallel to the phase-encoding axis. Inappropriate adjustment of the RF system can also produce artifacts.

In most MR imaging suites, a special enclosure, the Faraday cage, which is made of low-resistance metal such as copper or aluminum surrounds the room on all six sides and is responsible for keeping extraneous radio frequencies from entering the scan environment. The Faraday cage also includes RF enclosures about doors and windows. If the scan room door is left open during the imaging procedure, RF leaks can occur from outside the room, resulting in radio-frequency noise and artifacts. Any breach in the integrity of the Faraday cage can result in RF artifacts.

Solution

Meticulous operating techniques by the MRI personnel will result in a reduction in potential RF artifacts. This includes careful preparation by the MRI technologist so that the scan environment is free of any object that may produce radio frequency and thus the potential for artifacts. Table electronics and metering devices must be turned off during the scanning procedure to ensure optimal image quality. The door to the scan room should remain closed and secured during the imaging procedure. The patient should be scanned in clothing that does not have the potential for producing any artifacts. The best material is 100 percent cotton, and this clothing should be issued at the site.

Only direct current (DC) should be used in the scan room to eliminate the possibility of AC fluctuation, which can cause artifacts. This includes circuitry to electrical components used in the suite, and even the type of light bulbs. Electrical equipment that must reside in the room during the procedure must be adequately RF shielded.

Thorough system checks by service engineers should be performed at regular intervals to ensure that RF interference does not occur. If RF interference is suspected of causing artifacts, an easy method that the operator can use to check for this is to take a transistor radio into the imaging suite, secure the door, and attempt to obtain a radio signal. If a radio signal is successfully received, a loss in the integrity of the RF room has occurred. More sophisticated methods of performing systematized checks for RF leaks are available to the qualified service engineer; however, this tactic provides quick results.

Data Clipping Errors

Data clipping errors occur because the bandwidth of the A/D converter is insufficient, and therefore the converter is unable to handle a high signal for a given receiver gain attenuation value. Algorithmic errors then occur during reconstruction, and incorrect gray-scale values are assigned to pixels. The resulting image looks as if there has been a video reversal; black becomes gray or white, and white becomes black (see Fig. 6-13).

RF power level (transmit power) and receiver gain ("listening power") are adjusted to ensure that enough power has been used to flip the proton spins into the transverse plane and that the resultant signal return is strong. The receiver gain can be thought of as the volume control. If it is too low, the signal will not be heard; if it is too high, distortion will result. Usually these values are defaults in the MR system based on acquisition orientation, slice thickness, sequence type, and field of view of the coil. Occasionally, the body part examined for a particular coil size (and therefore "canned" values of RF power and receive gain) does not fit within the range of values used for the particular sequence. For example, if an ankle is placed in a head coil, whose RF and receiver gain values have been adjusted for normal head FOV dimensions of between 20 and 25 cm, the system does not see as much signal return but continues to use a receiver gain that was based on the volume of a normal-size head. In this case, data clipping artifacts will probably result. Clipping may also be a result of too much signal for which the gain value does not match, such as in obese patient imag-

ing. If several high frequencies are clipped, the image will contain significantly reduced spatial resolution and image quality.

Solution

Some MR systems allow *operator intervention* in RF power levels and receiver gain values so that selections can be made to deal with changes in the scanning process that may be unavoidable, such as scanning a small body part in a large coil. When scanning a smaller body part than the coil was designed for, receiver gain values may be reduced so that abnormally high frequencies will not be incorporated into the reconstruction process.

Coil selection is very important in reducing the possibility for data clipping. Coils are designed to accommodate a specific field of view: Head coils accommodate normal head size, body coils are large to cover more volume, and extremity coils are used to scan smaller body parts. RF power levels and receiver gains are adjusted to default to a specific range according to the size of the expected body part and the imaging sequence type (gradient echo or any partial flip sequence necessitates less RF power than a spin echo sequence, since fewer spins are being flipped), patient orientation, and slice thickness. The MR system can make internal adjustments for changes in any of the last three areas; however, it cannot know the actual size of the body part being placed in the coil. Selecting a coil that best fits the anatomic region being examined will help to ensure that correct RF power levels and receiver gains are being used.

Patient positioning is an often forgotten but extremely important function that, when performed correctly, will reduce many unwanted artifacts. The imaging coils have their own field of view (sometimes referred to as the *sweet spot*) for which the best overall SNR will be attained. This is a function of coil design. When the anatomic region is outside the coil's FOV, tuning procedures are not accurate. This is in addition to the possibility that aliasing artifacts will occur. Inaccuracy in the selection of RF levels and receiver gains by the imaging system can result in clipping errors as well as images with inhomogeneous signals (in areas of expected homogeneity). The patient must be positioned in the coil in a central orientation for best overall signal reception. If the patient has an anatomic feature, such as severe kyphosis, which prevents normal patient/coil orientation, steps should be taken to adjust the positioning of the patient so that the body part being imaged is as centrally located in the coil as possible. For example, this may require that the patient be placed in a semi-oblique position, with the head turned to one side and propped on a sponge, to accomplish optimal brain imaging (see Chap. 1).

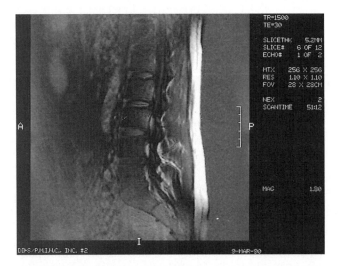

Figure 6-13 Image appears as if there has been a video black/white reversal.

If imaging a small body part in a large coil is unavoidable, taking steps to *load the coil* so that the receive coil sees more than is actually contained within will improve the chances that clipping will not occur. For large patients, use a coil that fully accommodates the body part without touching the patient.

Herringbone Artifact

This artifact gets its name from the fabric type it resembles (see Fig. 6-14). Other terms that have been used to describe the artifact are "corduroy" and "screen door." This artifact is particularly challenging in that it can have several possible origins, can be intermittent or consistent, subtle or conspicuous, and can present on one image or all images of a set.

Herringbone appearance has already been discussed under radio-frequency artifacts. Radio-frequency discrepancies in the system can cause electromagnetic spikes that are recovered and stored in the time domain during data acquisition. Therefore, the time-domain data contain erroneous information, which will be processed.

Surges in the gradient power can result in large spikes during data acquisition, resulting in herringbone artifacts.

Fluctuation of currents within the scan environment, such as old light bulbs in the room or alternating current for light bulbs, can cause herringbone artifact.

Solution

The appearance of this artifact necessitates *evaluation by the service engineer.* Raw (unprocessed) data saved by the MRI technologist will prove quite useful in diagnosing the problem.

Free Induction Decay (FID) Artifact

The FID artifact is a discrete type of artifact which appears edge to edge on the matrix in the frequency-encoding direction when excessive noise is inherent to the imaging system. It presents most often as a linear dashed line through the center of the encoding matrix with a centrally located bright or dark signal (see Fig. 6-15) and is sometimes referred to as the *zero-line, central point,* or *DC offset* artifact. It is very similar in appearance to some RF artifacts. Depending on signal processing, it may also appear as a "star" artifact, which has a bright signal only at the center of the slice.

The artifact is a result of remnant-free induction decay which follows the 180° refocusing pulse. The signal

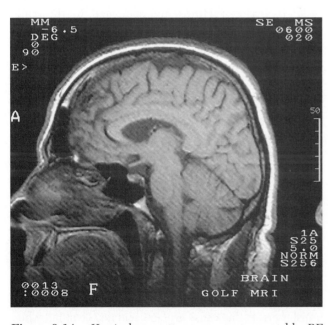

Figure 6-14   Herringbone pattern appearance caused by RF interference.

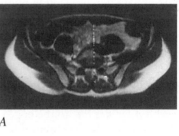

A

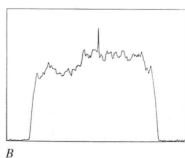

B

Figure 6-15   FID artifact seen as dashed line through center of image.

representing individual data sample points is obtained based on the contour of the sine function, which drops off rapidly on either side of the amplitude, or center point. Signals that fall within the normal range will be assigned an appropriate gray-scale value. Those signals representing high noise will have high amplitudes and persistent sidelobes of the sine wave, unlike the normal sidelobes, which are minimal. The dashed lines often associated with FID artifacts originate from the persistent sidelobes that align parallel to the frequency-encoding axis.[4]

The FID artifact may have several different origins. When it appears on a frequently used sequence, it can be a result of inappropriate adjustment or shift of the Y and $-Y$ phase waveforms. If the RF system is not adjusted properly, FID artifacts may be seen. Some sequences that are gradient-intensive, such as flow compensation and fast scan sequences, are very sensitive to imperfect adjustments of the RF system. If the amplitude ratio between the 90° and 180° pulses is different from the normal ratio, the artifact tends to be manifested.

FID artifact is more apparent when single or half acquisitions are used, since noise will not be averaged out of the final image.

Solution

This artifact occurs less frequently than in the early days of MRI as a result of the increased sophistication of most imagers. If an FID artifact is commonly seen, the problem could be due to excessive noise or inappropriate system adjustments, which the service engineer must evaluate.

Increasing the number of acquisitions can minimize the effect of the artifact because system noise is more apt to be averaged out of the final image.

The *DC offset* (phase cycling of the RF) can be adjusted by the service engineer; however, with time, it can drift back to the original position, producing the artifact.

Many manufacturers eliminate the problem caused by the artifact's position in the center of the image by *shifting the central reference line* to the edge of the matrix during display, where it will not obscure anatomic structures.

Partial Volume Effect

The partial volume effect occurs when different anatomic structures whose signals are heterogeneous are contained within the same pixel. During data reconstruction, the sig-

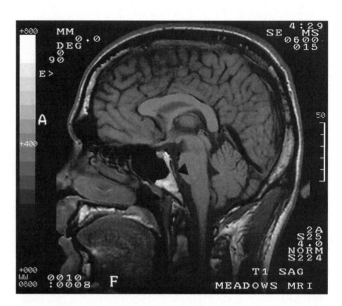

Figure 6-16 Sagittal brain shows partial volume effect as gray signal intensity within the dark CSF, identified by arrowhead.

nal from each voxel is averaged, and one gray-scale value is assigned to the resulting pixel. This gray-scale value is nonspecific if more than one signal is contained in the initial voxel of tissue. The resultant artifact is that of inhomogeneity of signal (see Fig. 6-16).

This artifact is more pronounced in regions of the body where there are large differences in tissue structures, such as the non-signal-producing sphenoid sinus adjacent to the bright pituitary. In this case, if the image is acquired as a thick slice or pixel size is large, both structures are contained in the same voxel, and the resulting gray-scale value is an average of both.

Solution

Partial volume effect can be eliminated or minimized by *using thinner slices* or by *reducing the pixel size* (smaller voxel volume) to acquire the data. The smaller the voxel, the more likely it is that one structure will be represented by the pixel.

Artifacts can be caused by circumstances other than those described above (see Figs. 6-17A and B and 6-18A and B). They can be caused by reconstruction errors, in which case the operator can try re-reconstructing the sequence in an attempt to remedy the situation. Image transfer errors that cause artifacts seldom occur, but when they do, they create an image that contains information from multiple sequences. *Warping* describes a distorted

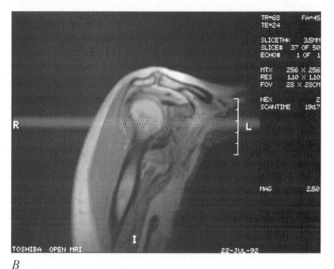

A

B

Figures 6-17 *A* and *B*. Reconstruction error which was resolved by re-reconstructing the image.

The Language of Artifacts

Aliasing   Superimposing objects outside of the field of view on the actual image.

Bleeding   Smearing of signal in a phase-encoding direction image; usually appears as unstructured signal in noise region.

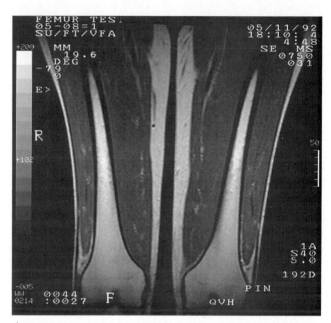

A

B

Figures 6-18 *A* and *B*. Warp artifact caused by coupling.

appearance and is seen commonly with metallic artifacts (see Fig. 6-18*A* and *B*). It can also occur when the patient's body part touches the coil and interference from the electric currents in the body produces magnetic susceptibility, which in turn creates the artifact. Finally, camera errors can produce unfinished, ragged, or distorted images (see Fig. 6-19).

This chapter is intended to be used as a reference in identifying the artifacts that are most commonly seen in MR imaging and over which the operator has reasonable control. Having become familiar with the origin of MR artifacts, the technologist can apply techniques and methods that will eliminate, at best, or reduce the potential for these artifacts.

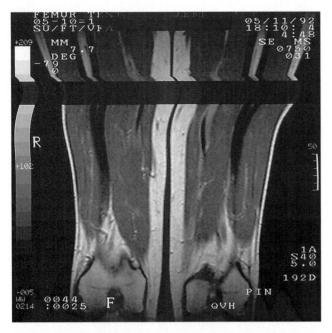

Figure 6-19   Laser camera error.

Blurring — Uneven edges and loss of detail; may be caused by motion, low-resolution imaging techniques, high filtration methods, or discontinuity in signal intensities, resulting in truncationlike artifacts.

Bright lines — Bright columns of pixels extending the height of the image; usually associated with single-frequency RF noise.

Clipping — Result of inappropriate RF power levels and receiver gains used to image an object with abnormally high or low signals; reconstruction errors result, with video reversal appearance in the image.

Dark lines — Black rows of pixels extending the width of the image; usually associated with damage of the disk data record.

Distortion — Image appears stretched, shrunk, or somewhat displaced from the true configuration; typically, straight lines appear as curves, or rectangles are displayed as parallelograms.

FID — Artifact from remnant "free induction decay" following 180° pulse; typically seen on second echo or one-acquisition images; appears as faint signal lines extending along center row of pixels.

Flares — Unusually bright signals in small, localized regions.

Freckles — Random pixels that display brighter than their neighbors even though they measure a smaller intensity of signal.

Fuzziness — Absence of crispness in the image; typical pixel display looks as if interpolation has already occurred.

Garbage — Degradation of the image that is so severe that the subject structure may not even be distinguished.

Ghosting — Faint inverted copy of the signal region is visible, nominally offset along a diagonal.

Herringbone — The image is overlaid with alternating lighter and darker bands which resemble the fabric pattern (i.e., closely packed triangular waveforms).

Magnetic susceptibility — The intensity of induced magnetization of an object that is exposed to an external magnetic field.

Missing signal — An image slice which should have a subject on it, has none; the data on the image are nonzero but are random noise.

Missing slices — An image slice is not recoverable; if it is recoverable, it contains no nonzero data.

Motion — The image subject appears replicated; this will be seen only in patient studies where physical motion of the subject occurs, such as respiratory and cardiac motion, blood flow, or voluntary repositioning of the patient.

Noise structure — A portion of the image which should contain random noise appears to contain patterns or structures.

Pixelation — Curved or diagonal edges display like stair steps because of discrete limit of image resolution.

Popcorn — Random intensely bright spots appearing scattered around the time-domain image, observable on images generated without Fourier transform; represents strong sporadic noise being injected into the receive path.

Replication — Similar to bleeding except that the structure of the signal region is perceptible in the noise region; sharp edges are visible.

RF inhomogeneity — The periphery of the subject is

	slightly brighter than the center because of its proximity to the RF coil antenna.
Ringing	Repetitious banding observed at the edges of the subject; may also be seen with faint replication of edge lines in noise region adjacent to true edge; also known as truncation or Gibbs artifact.
Squashed	The image appears compressed, vertically and/or horizontally.
Tilt	The image appears rotated from true alignment.
Walking	An object placed perpendicular to the imaging planes appears to shift diagonally in successive slices.
Warping	Distortion of the image resulting from field inhomogeneities or gradient instability.
Wraparound	Part of the image overlay appears on both sides of the image as a result of limitations of field of view and resolution; also known as aliasing.
Zipper	Nominally also viewed in time-domain images, zipper artifacts are seen as alternating bright and dark dashes across a row of pixels.

References

1. Stark DD, Bradley WG Jr: Artifacts, in *Magnetic Resonance Imaging.* St. Louis: Mosby, 1988.
2. Elster AD: MR artifacts, in *Questions and Answers in Magnetic Resonance Imaging.* St. Louis: Mosby, 1994.
3. Elster AD: MR artifacts, in *Questions and Answers in Magnetic Resonance Imaging.* St. Louis: Mosby, 1994.
4. Wheeler GL: Artifacts, in Woodward P, Freimarck R: *MRI for Technologists.* New York: McGraw-Hill, 1995.

Suggested Readings

Elster AD: *Questions and Answers in Magnetic Resonance Imaging.* St. Louis: Mosby, 1994.

Haacke EM, Bellon EM: Artifacts, in Stark DD, Bradley WG Jr: *Magnetic Resonance Imaging.* St. Louis: Mosby, 1988.

Wheeler, GL: Artifacts, in Woodward P, Freimarck R: *MRI for Technologists.* New York: McGraw-Hill, 1995.

Part II

Special Techniques

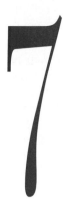

Fast Scan Techniques

Reducing the time required to collect the MR data improves scan time and increases patient compliance, which results in optimal image quality. This was realized shortly after the development of MRI technology. Fast scan imaging techniques are therefore not new to MR—techniques such as gradient/field echo imaging and conjugate symmetry have been used extensively in the past ten years. Using gradient reversal techniques to refocus spins allows a reduction in the flip angle of the RF pulse, so that T1 and T2 relaxation occur more rapidly. Because of this shortened T1 and T2 time, both TR and TE can be decreased. Narrow-bandwidth technology used in conjunction with conjugate symmetry imaging improves SNR, thereby allowing a reduction in the number of acquisitions. Although these methods permit reduced scan times, certain aspects of the technologies produce artifacts (magnetic susceptibility and increased chemical shift artifact) and/or loss of SNR (gradient echo imaging). As a result, investigation of other modes of fast scanning has been implemented. In the recent past, more sophisticated imaging techniques have been designed that have improved our ability to gather MR data in record time. Each scheme has its own useful application and should be chosen with care, based on clinical need. This chapter provides a conceptual framework for understanding fast scan techniques used in MRI today.

K Space

The foundation used to manipulate scan speed is contained mostly in the time-domain or raw data file. We call this file *k space,* and rely on its symmetry to allow us the pleasure of exploiting its contents. K space is acquired in a predictable manner as defined by the phase-encoding and frequency-encoding gradients. Each line of k space contains spatial and signal information for the entire image. In order to fully understand the mechanisms behind the more sophisticated fast scan techniques, we must comprehend the concept of k space and the manner in which it is filled.

K space can be thought of as a file folder that contains all the information about an image. It is acquired as a series of lines, as defined by the phase-encoding gradient. Each line contains a multitude of data sample points, or measured MR signal values that are obtained by data sampling (echo collection) during the frequency-encoding process (see Fig. 7-1).

Each line of k space contains all the information required to process an entire image. K space can contain a small or large amount of information which can be related to scan time (a low or high number of phase-encoding steps). All the information or only portions of the information may be used. In conventional spin echo and gradient echo imaging, all lines of k space are filled during the course of an acquisition and are used to produce the final image by Fourier transformation. In addition, each echo of the conventional sequence will have its own k-space file. For each repetition TR, the phase-encoding gradient is incremented, so that the echo is acquired with an altered phase and the next line in the k-space file is occupied (see Fig. 7-2). The process is repeated until k space is entirely filled.

The encoding gradients are pivotal about k space, so that an additional important property of k space is its symmetry. The values that are placed in the k-space data points correspond to the MR signal amplitudes at various

Phase encoding

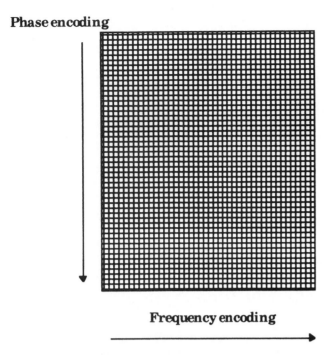

Frequency encoding

Figure 7-1 K space for one echo contains lines of data samples collected during the echo. The central portion of k space is about the center of both the lines of phase encoding and the data samples of frequency encoding.

times during the echo. Since the phase-encoding gradient is incremented for each repetition, the slope of the phase-encoding gradient corresponding to the top and bottom of k space is relatively high, whereas the center lines of k space correspond to a very small or zero slope of the gradient (see Fig. 7-3). The relationship of signal amplitude to phase increment based on gradient slope is such that the highest signal amplitude corresponds to the lowest phase-gradient slope. In other words, if the slope of the gradient is minimal, so that there is little or no gradient-induced dephasing, the signal will be the strongest. High gradient slopes result in increased phase dispersion and improved spatial resolution. Lower gradient slopes contribute to signal and contrast of the image.

In the usual method of k-space filling, the values on the left side of the rows (lines) of data are obtained early in the echo, and the values on the right side of the rows are obtained late in the echo collection. The center of k space corresponds to the center of the echo and contains the highest MR signal values. To reiterate, these central values are a result of high signal amplitude due to less gradient-induced dephasing as a consequence of minimal or zero gradient slope. Phase-encoding steps that have a positive gradient slope are mathematically related to those corresponding to the negative slope, so that theoretically only half the phase-encoding steps need be acquired. The rest can be interpolated. These concepts will become im-

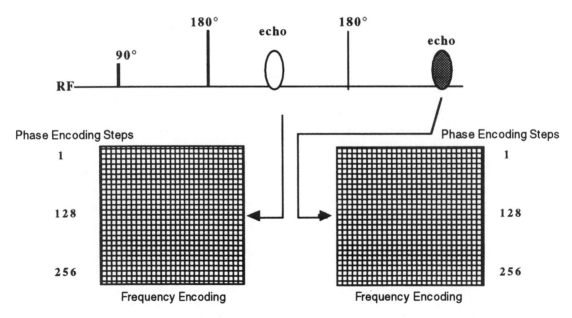

Figure 7-2 K-space filling for a dual-echo sequence; one line of k space is filled for each repetition. Each echo has its own k-space file.

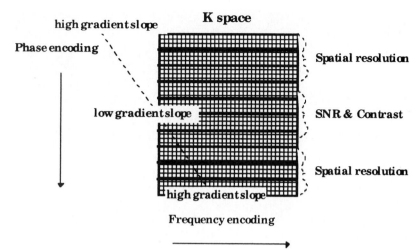

Figure 7-3 K-space phase-encoding gradient slope dependence on SNR, contrast, and spatial resolution.

portant in understanding the contrast and resolution control of data acquisition by fast scan techniques.

Fast Scan Imaging Techniques

Mechanisms that Shorten Overall Scan Time

Data acquisition time can be reduced either by acquiring the information more rapidly or by reducing the amount of data collected. The speed of data acquisition of an MRI is determined by several primary imaging factors: repetition time (TR), the number of phase-encoding steps (#PE), and the total number of times the data are acquired (N_{acq}). The number of 3D slices contributes to scan time when 3DFT imaging techniques are used. Using conventional spin echo imaging techniques, scan time can be decreased by reducing the *repetition time,* the *number of phase-encoding steps,* and/or the *number of data collection passes.* There are several disadvantages to changing one of these parameters as a method of reducing scan time: Decreasing TR reduces SNR and limits contrast; decreasing the number of phase-encoding steps reduces SNR by a square root factor and decreases spatial detail; decreasing the number of acquisitions reduces SNR by a square root factor and is usually limited by one.

Gradient or field echo imaging, by definition, realizes a reduced scan time by virtue of partial flip imaging techniques. Lowering the flip angle means that fewer spins are directed to the transverse plane, so that less time is

needed for longitudinal remagnetization (T1 recovery). As a result, TR can be reduced, lowering scan time, while maintaining the desired contrast using flip angle selections. The primary clinical application of gradient echo imaging using partial flip angles is to obtain T2-like contrast in short scan times. Further reductions in scan time by reducing the phase-encoding matrix or the number of acquisitions have potentially detrimental consequences, as mentioned above. The disadvantages of this technique are related to magnetic susceptibility effects, chemical shift artifact (phase cancellation), and limitations in echo times.

Another method by which fast scanning can be accomplished is by using a *variable-TR* imaging technique. This approach is based on the concept that signal and contrast information for an image are placed at the center of k space, where frequency amplitude is high. When the sequence is begun, a shorter TR is used than would normally be used for the desired contrast. As data collection continues, the TR is gradually increased until the TR that corresponds with the desired contrast is reached. The echo is sampled, and the signal values are placed in the middle segment of k space, which corresponds to the central phase-encoding steps. Following primary data collection, the TR is gradually dropped to a low point. The data points that correspond to the lowered TR time are associated with the periphery of k space, and therefore spatial resolution of the image (see Fig. 7-4). In this method, the scan time can be reduced by a factor that coincides with the average of the TR times used, usually 20 to 40 percent. A dual-echo set of images whose image contrast and signal are maintained or improved can be obtained without the usual increase in scan time. The clinical usefulness of variable-TR imaging is related to the production of images that have bright fluids without the disadvantages associated with gradient echo imaging. The number of slices available is limited by the lowest TR used; in comparison with conventional techniques, this is a disadvantage. In addition, a blurring effect may be noted if there is a large

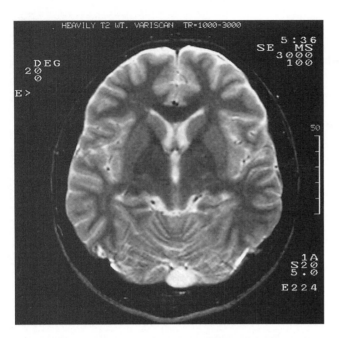

Figure 7-4 Variable TR image. (*Courtesy Toshiba America Medical Systems, Inc. By permission.*)

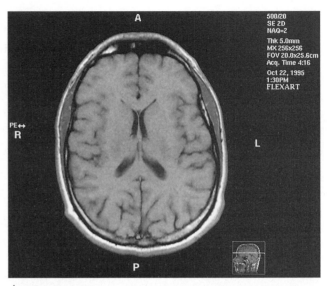

A

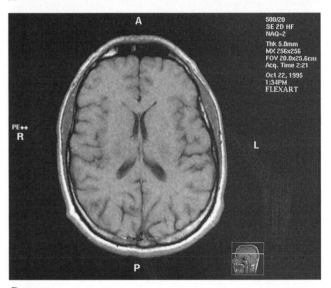

B

Figure 7-5 (*A*) Conventional transaxial brain using $2N_{acq}$; (*B*) an HFI image using $2N_{acq}$. (*Courtesy Queen of the Valley Hospital. By Permission.*)

difference between the shortest and the longest TR. This phenomenon is related to signal intensities and is similar to the truncation artifact (see Chap. 6).

Mechanisms that Reduce the Amount of Data Collected

The strategy of reducing the amount of data collected exploits the symmetry of k space by collecting only a portion of the data and filling in the rest, as is practiced with conjugate symmetry techniques. *Half-Fourier imaging* fits into this category of imaging schemes. Using half-Fourier imaging, only half the total number of phase-encoding steps are collected to create images. It is a way to break the "one-acquisition barrier." The clinical usefulness of half-Fourier imaging is in acquiring true proton- and T2-weighted brain images without the contrast or resolution compromises found with the use of other methods, and to provide a mechanism for acquiring breath-hold images of the abdomen.[1] The primary disadvantage is an overall loss in SNR as compared to conventional spin echo imaging (see Fig. 7-5).

Another scheme uses *matched-bandwidth technology* to collect slightly over half the data sample points (frequency-encoding steps) (see Fig. 7-6). The technology allows a reduction in the TE, an increase in overall SNR, if the bandwidth is reduced, and an increase in the total number of slices per TR. This technique has been shown to be quite advantageous at mid- and low field strengths for its improvement in signal-to-noise ratio. The primary disadvantages of matched-bandwidth imaging are its increased sensitivity to motion and increased magnetic sus-

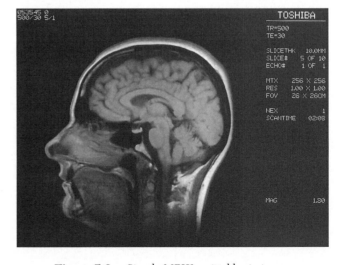

Figure 7-6 Simple MBW sagittal brain image.

TABLE 7-1 FAST SCAN IMAGING NOMENCLATURE

	GE	Philips	Picker	Siemens	Toshiba
Spin echo	Spin echo	Spin echo	Spin echo	Spin echo	Spin echo
Partial flip imaging	GRASS, SPGR	FFE	Field echo, FAST	FLASH, FISP	Field echo, PFI
Variable TR					VariScan
Half-Fourier imaging	Fractional NEX	Half-scan	Phase conjugate symmetry	Half-Fourier imaging	HFI
Matched-bandwidth imaging	Half-echo imaging	Optimized second echo	Read conjugate symmetry	Optimized bandwidth	MBW, Opt M
RARE	Fast spin echo	Turbo SE	Fast spin echo	Turbo spin echo	FastSE
Quadscan	POMP				QuadScan
Snapshot	Fast SPGR	Turbo FE	RAMFAST	Turbo FLASH	FastFE

Adapted from Winkler ML, Schwartz GM: Traversing k space with fast MR scans. MRI insights. *Diagnostic Imaging,* May 1994.

ceptibility effects. In addition, if the readout bandwidth is reduced in an effort to further improve SNR, some loss of resolution may be present as a result of increased chemical shift artifact.

Mechanisms that Reduce Scan Time by Filling K Space Rapidly

Fast spin echo and *fast gradient echo imaging techniques,* known by a variety of names, use modifications of conventional sequence schemes to acquire multiple data collection steps during a TR. In the methodology discussed up to this point, scan time was shortened by reducing specific scan parameters that directly relate to scan time, or by reducing the amount of data collected. Typical fast scan techniques that reduce scan time by filling k space rapidly do so by collecting data from *multiple echoes* during a repetition and using all the data to create *one or more* images. Table 7-1 shows common terminology used for fast scan techniques.

Fast spin echo, known generically as *RARE* imaging, uses the conventional spin echo pulse sequence in a modified manner to acquire all the lines of k space in a smaller amount of time. In conventional SE imaging, one line of k space for each echo is filled for each repetition (see Fig. 7-2). Scan time is based in part on the total number of lines of data contained within k space: 128, 256, etc. Each echo will have its own k-space file, whose data will be mathematically transformed during the Fourier process.

In fast spin echo imaging, each TR will be used to collect a multitude of data sample lines (phase-encode lines containing data sample information gathered from each echo), which will be placed into k space in groups or segments. The lines of data, which have been gathered from multiple echo samples, will be used to contribute to one final image (see Fig. 7-7). The speed at which k space is filled is defined by how many lines of data (how many echoes) fit into each group or segment. Scan time is therefore reduced by the number of echoes collected per TR.

In a conventional dual-echo SE sequence, a phase encoding is performed for each TR, so that each echo is

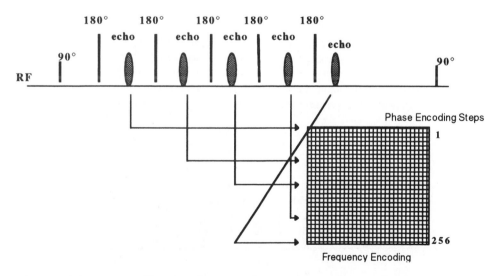

Figure 7-7 K space filling in a fast spin echo sequence. In this example, five echoes are collected during one TR, filling k space in one-fifth the normal time.

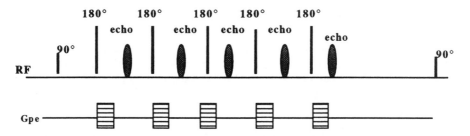

Figure 7-8 Each echo has its own phase-encoding gradient whose slope is incremented differently.

acquired with the same phase encoding, but the echoes are sorted into separate k-space files, line by line. Two images will be created, each with contrast that is unique to the echo times used.

Similar in design to the conventional spin echo pulse sequence, fast spin echo imaging is initiated using a 90° RF pulse. However, multiple echoes, preceded by successive 180° refocusing pulses prior to each echo sampling, are acquired for each repetition. A separate phase-encoding gradient is applied prior to each echo so that different lines of k space that correspond to the different echoes are filled (see Fig. 7-8).

Fast spin echo imaging techniques can acquire between three and several hundred echoes in one repetition. The echoes are referred to as *echo trains,* and the length of the echo train, known as *ETL,* will contribute to the scan time. Scan time in fast spin echo imaging is therefore the product of TR, #PE, and N_{acq}, divided by the ETL. The longer the ETL, the faster the data will be collected.

$$\text{Scan time (seconds)} = \frac{[\text{TR (seconds)} \times \#\text{PE} \times N_{acq}]/\text{ETL}}{60 \text{ (seconds)}}$$

Each echo represents a different line of k space that will be added to one k-space file instead of many files. This file will be transformed to create one image whose contrast is a mixture of all echoes in the echo train. This echo is known as the effective TE, or *ETE* (sometimes known as TE_{eff}). The contrast of the image is dependent on which echo is placed in the middle of k space. Recall that the center of k space contributes to the signal and the contrast of the resultant image, while the periphery re-

lates to spatial resolution. The effective echo is placed in the middle of k space and will be used along with all other echoes collected to create an image that has the desired contrast (see Fig. 7-9).

The time interval between successive echoes in an echo train will have an effect on the contrast of the image through its effect on T1 or T2 contribution. This time interval can be called *echo-train spacing,* or *ETS.* The size of the ETS will in part determine at what millisecond the last echo will be sampled. Fast spin echo sequences can have exactly the same ETE and ETL; however, if the ETS is different, the resultant contrast may be different because the last echo may have more T2 contribution to the contrast mix.

In the example shown in Fig. 7-10, the sequence whose fifth echo is sampled at 140 ms and whose first echo is sampled at 60 ms will contribute more T1 weighting to the ETE of 100 ms because of the earlier echo collection. It will also have less SNR as a consequence of the added T2 dephasing accompanied by the last sample. The size of the ETS also has an effect on coverage. When the echoes are spaced so that they take up a good portion of the repetition time, there is little available space to perform the functions needed for generating multiple slices. As a result, the number of slices per TR is reduced when the ETS is large.

The actual echo times that make up the echo train of a fast spin echo sequence will all contribute to the contrast of the image; however, the resultant signal-to-noise ratio and contrast for the image will be roughly comparable to those of a standard spin echo sequence. Depending on the time component of the first and last echoes as well

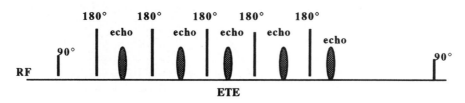

Figure 7-9 Effective TE identifies the effective contrast of the resultant image and corresponds to the echo whose signal information is placed in the middle of k space.

middle of k-space.

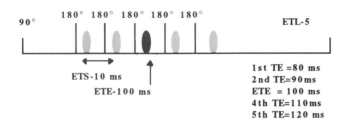

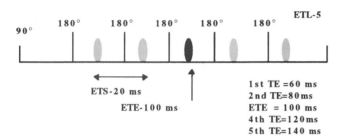

Figure 7-10 Effect of ETS on the position of the last echo of the echo train. This example shows two fast SE pulse sequence diagrams, both with an ETL = 5 and ETE = 100 ms.

as the echo spacing, the ETE may be more T1-weighted or T2-weighted than a conventional spin echo sequence with the same echo time. This concept is exemplified by the phenomenon of very bright signals seen in fat on T2-weighted fast spin echo sequences. This phenomenon is a consequence of heavy T1 contribution to the ETE as a result of data from more early echoes than late echoes being sampled. Many vendors have a variety of sequences with different ETL and ETE values and different echo-train spacing to provide the operator with a choice of contrast in the resultant image (see Fig. 7-11).

The most obvious benefit of using fast spin echo sequences is the dramatic reduction in scan time, especially when obtaining T2-weighted images. When high echo trains are used, the scan-time reduction is significant enough to allow an increase in scan-time parameters, resulting in more T2 contrast and improved signal. For example, in a conventional SE sequence where TR = 3000 ms, PE matrix = 256, and N_{acq} = 1, a respectable T2-weighted scan would be obtained in 12.8 min. Using the same scan parameters with a fast SE sequence of ETL = 15 yields similar results in less than one minute! We can improve on the image quality by increasing the TR to minimize T1 contrast, thereby improving T2 contrast, and increasing N_{acq} to increase SNR. Even if we use TR = 5000 ms and N_{acq} = 4, the scan time is still only 5.7 min, and the image produced is that of highly T2-weighted contrast.

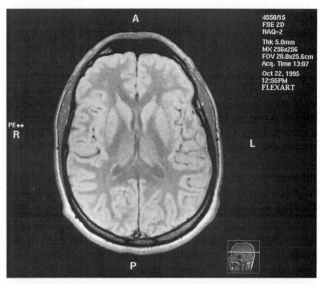

A

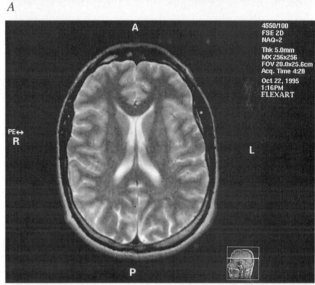

B

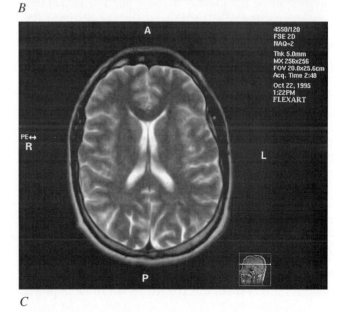

C

Figure 7-11 Images using (*A*) ETL = 3, (*B*) ETL = 9, and (*C*) ETL = 15. All other scan parameters are equal. (*Courtesy Queen of the Valley Hospital. By permission.*)

An added advantage of fast spin echo imaging is the minimization of magnetic susceptibility effects because of the use of repeated 180° RF pulses between echoes.[2] Recall that magnetic susceptibility effects are disadvantageous in most cases of gradient echo imaging. An example of a situation in which this effect may be desired is imaging for acute or chronic blood, both of which contain significant amounts of iron, which can be readily observed on most gradient echo images because of its magnetic susceptibility properties.

As is the case with MRI in general, there are some detrimental consequences of fast spin echo imaging. Any imaging technique that is gradient-intensive, such as fast spin echo, involves a reduction in the number of slices per TR. Since the gradients are using space that normally would be used to acquire additional slices, one cannot cover the same area that would have been covered using conventional SE techniques. In addition, the SAR (specific absorption rate) to the patient increases significantly with increasing ETL because of the added 180° RF pulses. Since every echo is sampled using a 180° refocusing pulse that is applied prior to data sample, the RF power deposition to the patient increases. SAR calculations are based on the weight of the patient and watts of power used in the RF pulse applications. These levels will increase when performing any RF-intensive imaging technique such as fast scan spin echo. If the patient is also large, SAR levels may increase dramatically. As a patient safety feature, most MRI vendors will automatically reduce the number of slices per TR to decrease calculated SAR levels. This further reduces coverage. Increasing the TR can help by allowing more time for tissue recovery after the last 180° pulse and echo collection so that more slices can be performed, increasing coverage. Decreasing the ETL can also reduce the patient SAR levels, allowing an increase in the number of slices per TR. In addition, when using fast scan techniques, the use of other RF-intense techniques, such as presaturation bands to minimize artifacts, can further increase RF power deposition to the patient, resulting in further reductions in the number of slices per TR. Prudent evaluation of system limitations with regard to patient size and RF-intense sequences, prior to initiating the scan, can minimize operator frustration.

An increase in ETL results in sequentially higher echoes being sampled to produce the contrast of the final image. This adds more T2 contrast to the mix in producing the image of specific ETE. The further out the last echo of the echo train, the more highly T2-weighted the image. If the echo-train spacing is wide, the last echoes contribute even more to the T2 mix. Because of additional T2 dephasing effects, the SNR is decreased for the ETE when using increased echo-train lengths. When the use of long ETL is desired, this phenomenon can be improved by decreasing the ETS, if this is possible on the system being used, so that the last echo is not as far out in time.

In addition, when the ETS is kept to a minimum, the number of slices per TR will increase.

Increased T1 contrast mix can give fat a very high signal on T2-weighted images. This can result from using a large ETL in which the first several echoes are very early in the train. Decreasing the contrast mix by shortening the ETL, so that the first echo is sampled later than the increased T1 contribution would allow, minimizes bright signal from fat on the T2-weighted image. However, with every late echo that is sampled, an additional T2 dephasing component will be added, which will lower SNR.

The last important disadvantage associated with fast spin echo techniques is related to the length of the echo train and the echo-train spacing. Since T2 decay continues throughout the sequence, the signal obtained from the last echo will be much weaker than those collected early on. The more echoes in the ETL, the greater the appearance of this signal difference. As a result, the Fourier transform may generate errors in signal registration, much like those seen when there is a large signal discontinuity between tissues, such as the cortex of bone and its fatty marrow. In conventional SE imaging, we call the artifact that is produced *truncation*. In fast SE, its appearance is more blurred, and may be misinterpreted as patient motion. Decreasing the ETL or ETS will minimize this artifact by decreasing the amount of signal difference. The consequence is an increase in scan time and/or lessened contrast mix.

Advanced fast spin echo imaging techniques are being developed that use spin echo refocusing technology (180° RF spin phase refocusing) for echo planar type acquisition. We can call these techniques *spin echo EPI*. Scan times for these sequences are often less than 1 s per image. Ultrarapid data acquisition results in significantly reduced motion artifacts. In addition, breath hold can be employed to virtually eliminate respiratory motion. Improvement of image quality using spin echo EPI techniques can be dramatic for applications in which high-T2-weighted contrast is desired or when functional imaging, diffusion imaging, or dynamic studies of various organs are desired (see Fig. 7-12).

The concept of echo planar imaging (EPI) is based on ultrafast data acquisition, with k space filled by rapid gradient reversals and echo collection after a single set of RF pulses.[3] The original design uses gradient-reversal techniques. However, it is plagued by limitations caused by hardware requirements (bigger and faster gradient coils, rapid-rate A/D converters, and increased computer memory), artifacts (increased chemical shift and eddy currents), acoustic noise (due to the increase in gradient vibration), and program flexibility.

Spin echo EPI was developed to counteract these limitations. It uses RF refocusing pulse technology, and so it is not limited by gradient power, does not produce the artifacts associated with eddy currents and chemical shift, and does not generate as much acoustic noise. As a result,

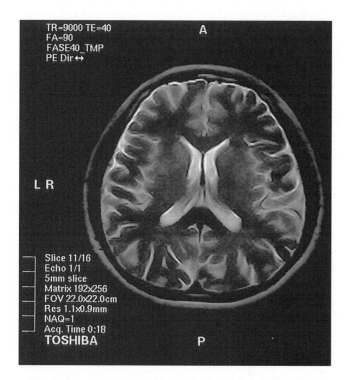

TR=9000 TE=40
FA=90
FASE40_TMP
PE Dir ↔

A

L R

Slice 11/16
Echo 1/1
5mm slice
Matrix 192x256
FOV 22.0x22.0cm
Res 1.1x0.9mm
NAQ=1
Acq. Time 0:18
TOSHIBA

P

Figure 7-12 Transaxial brain T2-weighted image using fast EPI spin echo technology. The entire scan was obtained in 18 s. (*Courtesy Toshiba America Medical Systems, Inc. By permission.*)

spin echo EPI has better contrast with fewer artifacts. Methods of producing the images using 2DFT or 3DFT allow for multislice images in seconds or high-resolution images, respectively (see Fig. 7-13).

Potential disadvantages of the technique include RF power deposition and increased SAR levels to the patient. Additionally, scan time is longer than for its gradient echo counterpart; however, the benefits of the sequence outweigh the minimal time increase.

Fast spin echo imaging is being relied on more and more as manufacturers and clinicians move down the learning curve with time and experience. Rapid imaging can be performed to produce highly T2-weighted images in record time, so that the technique has clinical utility in all applications where high T2 contrast is required. In addition, the dramatic savings in scan time can allow increases in scan parameters that directly affect SNR and resolution to further improve image quality (see Table 7-2).

Fast gradient echo imaging, known also as *snapshot imaging,* is essentially a modification of standard field echo imaging in which gradient reversals produce the echo. In the fast versions of this technique, image acquisition is performed with the shortest possible TR/TE combination to produce many echoes in an extremely short time (see Fig. 7-14). Because of the use of an ultrashort TR and TE, contrast control by the usual method is lost. This is compensated for by using various methods such as

a preparation pulse, reordering of k-space filling, and/or segmentation of k space.

In the simplest version of fast gradient echo imaging, the sequence is initiated with a preparation pulse followed by a waiting period referred to as the TI, similar to that used for inversion recovery imaging (see Fig. 7-15). Several gradient echoes are produced in rapid succession to acquire the image data, followed by a delay period before the pulse is repeated. Generally, the TI times used are on the order of 200 to 1000 ms with a repetition time of 9 to 13 ms. The repetition time remains very short, and so contrast control becomes a function of how soon data acquisition will occur following the inverting pulse and TI. This becomes a crucial component in the prediction and contrast control of the image.

Since the sequence involves the use of a 180° inverting pulse, contrast is similar to that seen in conventional IR sequences and is highly T1-weighted. Thus, the contrast curve for the sequence will have a familiar appearance, with complete inversion of the signal followed by gradual longitudinal recovery. As is the case with IR imaging, recovery is dictated by the T1 relaxation times for different tissues (e.g., that of fat is much less than that of water), so that the contrast components of separate tissues may be controlled through proper control of the time at which the echoes are generated (see Fig. 7-16). The TI chosen will also determine at what time data acquisition will occur, as it must be performed within a very small range of repetition times (typically between 9 and 13 ms). TI, therefore, is the parameter that ultimately defines the contrast of the image.

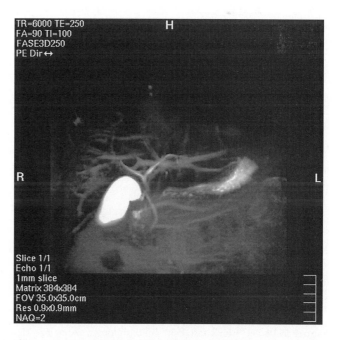

TR=6000 TE=250
FA=90 TI=100
FASE3D250
PE Dir ↔

H

R

L

Slice 1/1
Echo 1/1
1mm slice
Matrix 384x384
FOV 35.0x35.0cm
Res 0.9x0.9mm
NAQ=2

Figure 7-13 Coronal MR generated cholangio-pancreatography using 3DFT fast spin echo EPI. (*Courtesy Toshiba America Medical Systems, Inc. By permission.*)

TABLE 7-2 IMAGE OPTIMIZATION FOR FAST SPIN ECHO IMAGING

Scan Parameter	Action	Effect on Sequence	Explanation	Artifacts
TR	Increase	Increases SNR	Increases longitudinal magnetization	
(repetition time)		Increases T2W	Minimizes T1 contrast	
		Increases number of slices allowed	Increased TR	
		Increases scan time	Increased TR	Motion/flow
ETE (effective echo time)	Increase	Increases T2W	Maximizes T2 decay	
		Decreases SNR	Increased T2 decay	
ETL (echo train length)	Increase	Increases contrast mix	Increased number of echoes and variation	
		Reduces scan time	K space filled more quickly	
		Decreases number of slices allowed	Increase in late echo time	
		May increase blurring	Larger signal differences	Blurring
ETS (echo train spacing)	Decrease	Increases contrast control	First and last echo closer to ETE	
		Increases number of slices allowed	Decrease in late echo time	
		Decrease in blurring	Reduces signal jumps in k space	
PE steps (phase encoding)	Increase	Increases spatial resolution	Smaller pixel size; increased contrast	
		Decreases SNR/voxel	Smaller voxel volume	Pixel appearance
		Decreases truncation	Reduces tissue signal intensity differences	
		Increases scan time	ST = TR × #PE × NA	Motion/flow
		Increases SNR overall	Increases by √	
NA (number of acquisitions)	Increase	Increases SNR by √	Increased noise averaging	
		Increases scan time	ST = TR × #PE × NA	Motion/flow

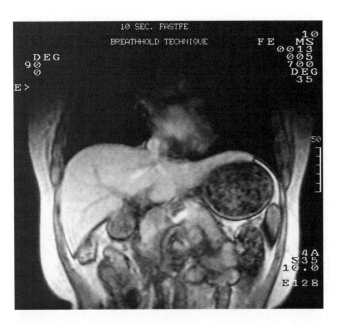

Figure 7-14 Coronal fast field echo abdomen using breath hold. (*Courtesy Toshiba America Medical Systems, Inc. By permission.*)

As in IR imaging, the TI represents the amount of time the net magnetic vector is allowed to recover T1 growth prior to data acquisition. The difference lies in the fact that only one line of data is acquired with each inversion pulse in IR imaging, whereas the entire image information is acquired for each inversion pulse in fast gradient echo imaging. The use of a short TI will have the effect of moving data acquisition so that it occurs earlier in the recovery process (see Fig. 7-17).

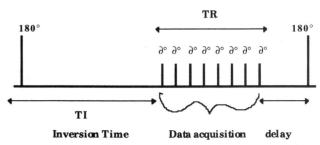

Figure 7-15 Simple fast gradient echo pulse sequence diagram using preparation pulse scheme.

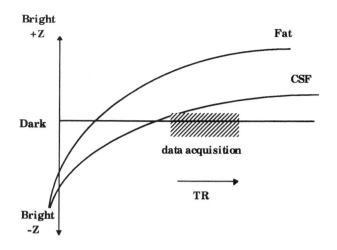

Figure 7-16   Contrast curve for fast gradient echo imaging.

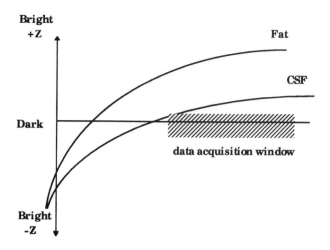

Figure 7-18   Effect of longer TI time.

If the TI is sufficiently short and data occur at about the null point of fat, it is possible to acquire data with little or no signal from fat, similar to the results achieved with the STIR technique. The difficulty here is that since you are acquiring several data lines in one pass, data acquisition (TR) must be adequate to collect all necessary data, so that specific contrast control is lost. For example, tissues that have short T1 recovery times and whose signals have been voided (they have crossed the null point on their way to longitudinal recovery when data acquisition occurs) are often mixed to produce the final image.

Increasing the TI will result in data acquisition that occurs late in the repetition. This can result in an increase in the signal obtained from both fat and water. Even though intermediate TI times of approximately 400 to 600 ms may provide sufficient contrast in the image, it is often recommended that the TI be increased to 700 or even 1000 ms to maximize the signal. Increasing the TI can affect scan time because TR must be increased to accommodate the change. This is contrary to the original objec-

tive of producing rapid T1-weighted images (see Fig. 7-18).

In fast gradient echo imaging, we are dealing with very short repetition times, so that signal-to-noise ratio and T1 contrast benefits are relatively small if the TR is increased. Additionally, an increase in TR will force an increase in the time at which data acquisition occurs following the inverting pulse, relative to TI (see Fig. 7-19).

When the time it takes to acquire the data is increased, more contrast changes occur over the period of the data acquisition. That is, the fat and water signals have more time to change relative to each other between the start of data collection and when it is finished. Therefore, increasing TR decreases contrast control at the expense of a minimal increase in scan time. It provides borderline improvements to SNR.

In fast gradient echo imaging, manipulating the TE will influence the contrast of the resultant image, but not

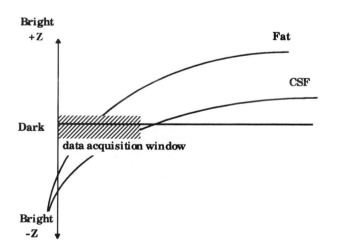

Figure 7-17   Effect of shorter TI time.

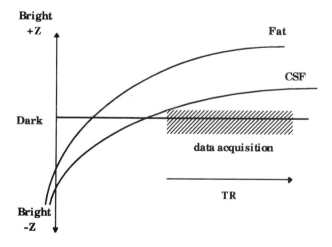

Figure 7-19   An increase in TR causes an increase in the time it takes to acquire the data, with a concomitant loss in contrast control.

to the extent it would with conventional imaging techniques. The primary goal of fast field echo imaging is to achieve a T1-weighted scan with good signal-to-noise ratio in a very short time. If TE is increased, a consequent forced increase in TR will be necessary, pushing out the time at which data acquisition occurs. As stated above, an increase in TR results in a loss of contrast control. It is advisable, then, to use the lowest possible TE available which results in an effective increase in the degree of T1 weighting as well as improved signal for this imaging technique. If a specific pathologic condition exists such that susceptibility effects can be beneficial in increasing the conspicuity of the lesion(s), the TE may be increased to provide out-of-phase chemical shift images (see Chap. 10).

In standard gradient echo imaging, decreasing the flip angle results in flipping fewer spins into the transverse plane, so that the T1 relaxation time is shortened. This allows a consequent shortening of both TR and TE, thus reducing scan time. The relationship between TR and flip angle is unique in conventional imaging, so that the number of spins flipped and the time allowed for their recovery have an impact on signal and contrast. In fast gradient echo imaging, the TR and TE are already ultrashort, so that the ability to vary the flip angle to control signal and contrast is lessened.

Finally, some general rules regarding phase-encoding selections must be offered. Increasing the PE will result in an increase in scan time as a result of the number of functions to be performed. When data acquisition is moved further out with respect to the sequence timing chart, contrast control is lessened. Therefore, using the minimum matrix resolution required to obtain the clinical information is advisable. If high-resolution imaging is necessary, the matrix may necessitate an increase; if resolution is not a priority, such as when performing kinematic or dynamic imaging, a reduced matrix may be selected. Every situation will be different, and so shrewd evaluation of diagnostic needs is required.

The order in which k space is filled significantly affects the resultant image contrast and is dictated by the limitations of the system hardware and software. It is not commonly operator-selectable for this reason. It generally is prioritized from one end to another in conventional imaging techniques. However, in fast gradient echo schemes, where the scan repetition times are very, very short, it is difficult to predict exactly where data collection occurs about each echo. In fast gradient echo imaging, it may in fact be advisable to begin data sample placement at the middle of k space and work to the periphery, in an attempt to ensure that the information that will contribute the most to contrast is actually recorded as such.

Contrast control can be improved by a method that is similar to the fast spin echo technique, where each echo is placed into a separate segment of k space. In fast gradient echo imaging, the data acquisition itself contains segments of echoes that are acquired over the entire sequence, including the preparation pulse. The scan is repeated many times, so that the segments are placed into k space sequentially until it is entirely filled. When the TI is kept constant, data acquisition occurs over a narrow range, with the net effect being a dramatic improvement in contrast control (see Fig. 7-20).

Each segment is placed in a predictable area of k space, so that contrast control improves because the relationship of frequency placement is known. K-space segmentation does increase scan time, however, as the entire sequence is repeated until all segments are filled.

Fast gradient echo imaging is used to collect data in the shortest time possible. This is partly accomplished by

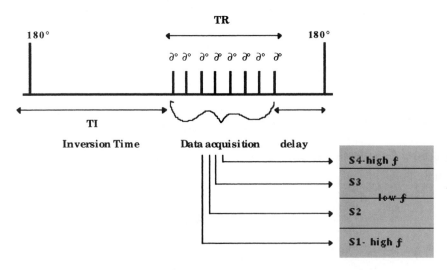

Figure 7-20 Fast gradient echo with segmentation. The entire pulse sequence is repeated (four times in this example), so that the data are placed into four segments of k space.

using ultrashort TR/TE combinations at the expense of contrast control. The resultant image contrast is very similar to that of the highly T1-weighted images seen using inversion recovery techniques and is manipulated using TI times (see Fig. 7-21).

As a consequence of the extremely short imaging times, this technique can produce multiple high-resolution T1-weighted thin-slice images for neurologic and musculoskeletal evaluation. It is also quite useful for imaging the abdomen and pelvis using breath-hold techniques, or when dynamic or kinematic studies are desired. MR myelographic studies where the CSF is brighter than the disk can be obtained, improving diagnostic capabilities in anatomic regions such as the cervical spine. Used in conjunction with contrast agents, fast gradient echo imaging can be used to evaluate heart perfusion and flow dynamics. Each clinical situation must be evaluated with care so that the sequence can be optimized for the diagnostic needs (see Table 7-3).

An elaboration of fast gradient echo imaging techniques was developed by Dr. Mansfield in the 1980s,

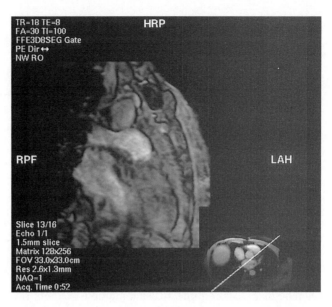

Figure 7-21 Fast field echo image of the coronary artery; scan time is 52 s. (*Courtesy of Toshiba America Medical Systems, Inc. By permission.*)

TABLE 7-3 IMAGE OPTIMIZATION FOR FAST GRADIENT/FIELD ECHO IMAGING

Scan Parameter	Action	Effect on Sequence	Explanation
TR (repetition time)	Decrease	Increase in contrast control	Decrease in data acquisition window
		Decrease in SNR	Marginal effect to very short initial TR
		Decreases scan time	Decrease in data acquisition window
TE (echo time)	Decrease	Improves contrast control	Due to shorter data acquisition window
		Decreases scan time	Allows reduced TR and less data acquisition
		Increases T1 contrast	General relaxation physics
		Increases SNR	Less T2° effects
PE steps (phase encoding)	Decrease	Decreases spatial resolution	Larger pixel size
		Increase in contrast control	Decrease in data acquisition window
		Increases SNR/voxel	Larger voxel volume
		Increase in truncation	Increases tissue signal intensity differences
		Decreases scan time	ST = TR × #PE × NA
FA (flip angle)	Increase or decrease	Direct effect on SNR by increase or decrease in number of spins directed to transverse plane	
		Small variation in FA which affects contrast allows little control	
TI (inversion time)	Increase	Increases SNR	Increase in T1 recovery
		Increase in T1 contrast	Data acquisition window to far right of contrast curve
		Increases scan time	Increase in time from inverting pulse to data acquisition
Delay (relaxation delay)	Increase	Increases SNR	Increased T1 growth after data acquisition
		Increases scan time	Increase in time required for all events
NA (number of acquisitions)	Increase	Increases SNR by √	Increased noise averaging
		Increases scan time	ST = TR × #PE × NA

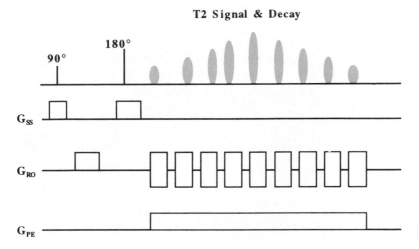

T2 Signal & Decay

Figure 7-22   EPI pulse sequence diagram.

when he demonstrated that by using multiple gradient reversals following *one set* of RF pulses, data acquisition and subsequent collection could be accomplished in subsecond imaging time. This concept was dubbed *echo planar imaging, or EPI.*

The original method of echo planar imaging makes use of ultrarapid gradient reversals to generate images (see Fig. 7-22). However, there are limitations caused by additional hardware and software requirements and artifacts related to chemical shift and eddy currents.

Another important consideration in echo planar imaging is related to the time-varying magnetic fields and subsequent induced currents associated with gradient magnetic field application. The amount of induced current in the patient's body depends on many factors. One of these factors is the rate of change, so that the faster and stronger the gradient magnetic field, the higher the expected induced current. EPI techniques routinely involve significant rates of change of gradient field, which could provoke much larger induced electric currents. The physiological effects that might result from current induction include but are not limited to neural or muscular stimulation, ventricular fibrillation, seizures, visual sensations, and changes in bone healing. For this reason, the use of these techniques on some patients may be precluded.[4]

The limitations associated with EPI have prompted the development of other sources of echo planar imaging. One, discussed above under fast spin echo techniques, uses rapid RF refocused pulses to generate the planar images. Other sources are currently being investigated, such as hybrids of gradient echo and spin echo technology involving multiple echoes, each with a different phase-encoding step, and multishot EPI, in which only gradient echo data are acquired using multiple acquisitions. The objective is to produce as many images as possible in split-second time with the fewest artifacts and the least detrimental effect on the patient (see Fig. 7-23). Compromises are thus being made that minimize chemical shift and magnetic susceptibility artifacts and induced electric cur-

rent (by use of spin echo technology) and still generate fairly rapid images (by using gradient echo technology).

The clinical application of echo planar imaging is quite varied. It includes functional imaging of the vital organs, such as the brain and heart (see Chap. 11), dynamic studies of the heart and GI tract, and diffusion imaging.

Quadscan is a fast imaging technique that can excite two or more separate slices simultaneously by using a composite RF pulse. The signal from this complex RF pulse is placed in k space which has an internally (not operator-selectable) doubled phase-encoding FOV. The RF pulses are phase-offset from one another, so that each im-

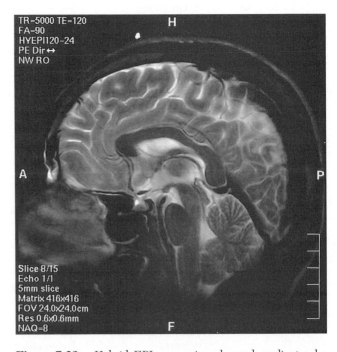

Figure 7-23   Hybrid EPI uses spin echo and gradient echo technology to produce high-resolution images of the brain. (*Courtesy Toshiba America Medical Systems, Inc. By permission.*)

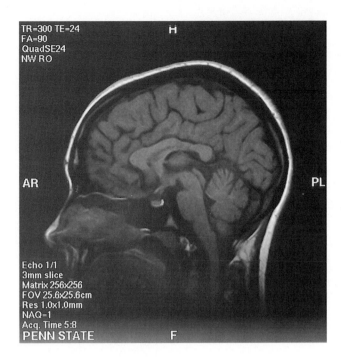

TR=300 TE=24
FA=90
QuadSE24
NW RO
H
AR
PL
Echo 1/1
3mm slice
Matrix 256x256
FOV 25.6x25.6cm
Res 1.0x1.0mm
NAQ=1
Acq. Time 5:8
PENN STATE
F

Figure 7-24   QuadScan field echo image of knee. (*Courtesy Toshiba America Medical Systems, Inc. By permission.*)

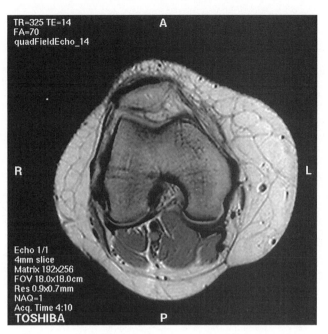

TR=325 TE=14
FA=70
quadFieldEcho_14
A
R
L
Echo 1/1
4mm slice
Matrix 192x256
FOV 18.0x18.0cm
Res 0.9x0.7mm
NAQ=1
Acq. Time 4:10
TOSHIBA
P

Figure 7-25   QuadScan spin echo image of brain. (*Courtesy Toshiba America Medical Systems, Inc. By permission.*)

age is encoded over a different range of phase encoding (0 to 360°) for later separation. The data contain information for separate images with preservation of spatial resolution.

Variations of this sequence, such as POMP (phase-offset multiplanar), produce two separate slices per TR. Quadscan (refer to Table 7-1) produces four slices per TR and does not increase the SAR. The advantage of this technique is its ability to acquire multiple T1-weighted images with true spin echo contrast.[5] Since the number of slices per TR is increased, repetition time can be shortened while allowing better T1 contrast control. The potential to improve SNR by increasing the number of acquisitions without a time penalty also exists. Currently, quadscan techniques can be employed using spin echo or gradient reversal techniques with similar advantages (see Figs. 7-24 and 7-25).

Fast scan imaging techniques are more popular than ever. These techniques have seen a dramatic improvement over the last several years that has helped to bolster confidence in their use. With further improvements and

technological advances, we should hope to reap the benefits with regard to image quality and acquisition time in the very near future.

References

1. Winkler ML, Schwartz GM: Traversing k space with fast MR scans. MRI Insights. *Diagnostic Imaging*, May 1994.
2. Winkler ML, Schwartz GM: Traversing k space with fast MR scans. MRI Insights. *Diagnostic Imaging*, May 1994.
3. Elster AD: *Questions and Answers in Magnetic Resonance Imaging*. St. Louis: Mosby, 1994.
4. Kanal E, Shellock FG: Safety considerations prevent harm in MRI. *MR*, May/June 1993.
5. Winkler ML, Schwartz GM: Traversing k space with fast MR scans. MRI Insights. *Diagnostic Imaging*, May 1994.

8

MR Vascular Imaging

Vascular imaging using MR technology has developed rapidly within the past several years to become a tool that is quite common in diagnostic imaging. Compared to early versions of MR vascular images, where image quality, resolution, and specificity were lacking, the images of today show significant improvement. This is generally a result of better gradient systems, more suitable pulse sequences, and the experience of the imaging team.

Although early investigation favored high-field-strength vascular imaging (because of a predominance of high-field-strength systems at research sites), the basic principles of MR vascular imaging are not dependent on field strength. Even though high field strength results in more intrinsic signal, it is also restricted by dephasing and susceptibility effects, increased motion sensitivity, and closer T1 tissue values between blood and stationary tissues[1] (see Fig. 8-1).

As we become more sophisticated regarding MR, we realize that it is imperative to consider the basis of the MR vascular techniques as related to the patient's clinical status before selecting an appropriate technique. Taking the time to optimize the technique based on the clinical indication and the patient's tolerance can produce optimum image quality.

MR vascular imaging techniques are developed to enhance the signal from blood while reducing the signal from background tissue. The factors that must be considered when choosing an MR vascular imaging technique are blood flow pattern, vessel geometry, and flow direction and velocity. Acquisition techniques that best demonstrate the structures of interest can then be optimized. Table 8-1 summarizes these effects.

Gradient Phase Effects

Spins that align in the same direction with respect to one another are said to be in phase; that is, they have a phase coherence because their phase angles are equal. The greater the phase coherence, the stronger the signal return. The net signal received by a coil will diminish if the phases begin to disperse, so that they lose phase coherence. The signals essentially cancel one another. Loss of phase coherence is a normal consequence of MRI and is a result of T2* effects from magnetic field inhomogeneities, chemical shift, magnetic susceptibility, and intrinsic T2 relaxation. In conventional imaging, compensatory gradients in the form of gradient reversals are designed to minimize the effects of phase dispersion for stationary spins by refocusing the phases after T2*. However, for moving spins, this becomes much more difficult to achieve.

Gradient waveforms are designed to correct for phase dispersion by incorporating a bipolar pulse. This pulse consists of two lobes with equal strength but opposite polarity. For stationary spins, this correction works quite well. For spins that move in the direction of the bipolar pulse, such as vascular flow, however, complete rephasing is not achieved, resulting in loss of signal within the vascular structure. In addition, artifacts from signal misregistration due to the moving spins are evident. Pulse sequence design can become quite sophisticated when the objective is to visualize signal in moving spins. It is suggested that the reader review and comprehend the concepts of gradient moment nulling techniques, described in detail in

69

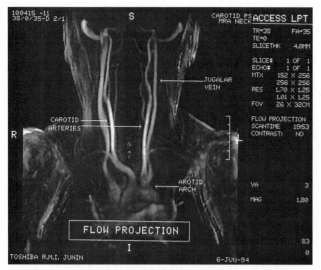

A

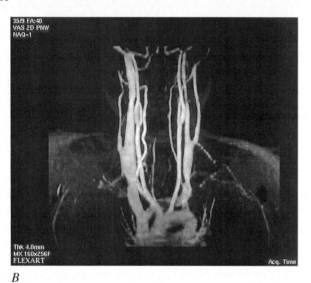

B

Figure 8-1 MR vascular image of carotid arteries at (A) 0.064 T and (B) 0.5 T. (*Courtesy Toshiba America Medical Systems, Inc. By permission.*)

Chap. 12, as flow compensation is an integral component of many vascular methodologies.

MR Vascular Imaging Techniques

MR vascular imaging techniques can be categorized by the primary method by which they produce vascular contrast. The purpose of this chapter is to review the major

MR vascular techniques used in clinical imaging, understanding that these techniques are merely combinations of basic sequences that are performed every day. Vascular sequences can take advantage of 2DFT or 3DFT technology. Gradient or field echo imaging techniques are used in conjunction with presaturation and flow compensation techniques to provide the best overall vascular signal intensity with the least amount of background signal, in a reasonable scan time. Gradient echo imaging uses a gradient reversal technique that is not slice-selective to refocus spins. The nonselective refocusing prevents the spins from experiencing loss of signal as a result of normal dephasing. The use of gradient echo technology also allows reduction in TR and TE, which helps to accentuate the vascular signal by reducing saturation of spins and dephasing effects.

Fat-suppression methods are used with increasing frequency to eliminate signal from short-T1 tissues that may simulate vascular enhancement. In addition, some investigators make use of the increased signal intensity afforded by paramagnetic injection (which also shortens T1 relaxation times). Care must be taken when imaging vascular structures with the use of paramagnetic agents, as enhancement can occur for *all* vessels, even if presaturation bands have been used. The signal from normally enhancing structures, such as the postcontrast pituitary, can also interfere with signal from vessels.

The techniques commonly used in clinical practice give a physiologic record of blood flow by either background suppression methods or background subtraction methods. The two fundamental approaches, time of flight (TOF) and phase contrast (PC), or phase shift imaging (PSI), offer different ways of acquiring the data, and each has clinical applications for which it is best suited.[2]

TABLE 8-1 FACTORS THAT AFFECT MR SIGNAL IN BLOOD VESSELS

Increased	Decreased
Low velocity	High velocity
Laminar flow	Turbulent, vortex flow
Gradient moment nulling (flow compensation)	Presaturation
Even-echo rephasing	Odd-echo rephasing
Acquisition with one slice	Multislice acquisition
Flow perpendicular to imaging plane	Flow parallel to plane
End slices closest to entry of blood flow	Slices furthest from flow entry
Gating	
Gadolinium	

Source: Elster AD: *Questions and Answers in Magnetic Resonance Imaging.* St. Louis: Mosby, 1994.

Background Suppression Techniques with Flow-Related Enhancement

This technique, better known as "time-of-flight" enhancement (TOF), uses 3DFT or multiple 2DFT data acquisitions to produce a vascular image. Saturation of stationary spins within the imaged volume by fast, repetitive radiofrequency pulses prevents recovery of longitudinal magnetization, so that the nonmoving spins produce little signal. Selected moving spins (arterial or venous) that are entering the imaging volume and have not received an RF pulse exhibit an "inflow" effect, resulting in vascular enhancement. Postprocessing ray tracing using maximum projection intensity (MIP) methods extracts the vessel tree from the data set to produce an angiographic appearance of the vessel without the use of invasive contrast injection.

Presaturation is commonly used to help prevent signal from opposing flow from interfering with the signal representing the desired vascular structure (see Fig. 8-2). Refer to Chap. 12 for a description of presaturation techniques. A region adjacent to the imaging volume receives an RF pulse prior to each excitation, so that signal from spins flowing into the volume will be suppressed.

Flow-compensated gradient echo imaging offers increased reliability in flow-related enhancement of moving spins, as described in Chap. 12.

Time-of-flight imaging techniques have a number of attractive features. Their inherent sensitivity to flow in any direction allows a single acquisition to be performed, so that misregistration or interference from undesirable mo-

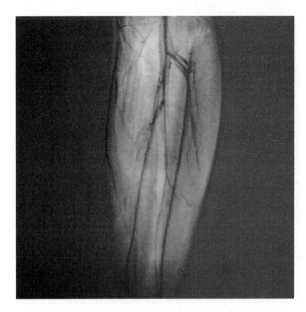

Figure 8-3   Peripheral vessels imaged with 2D TOF method.

tion does not occur as it can when subtraction methods such as phase shift are used. MR vascular imaging using TOF has low susceptibility to pulsatility and turbulence, reducing artifact potential. Additionally, image acquisition times can be relatively short, and the simplicity of the technique allows easy implementation and adjustment. The major disadvantages include a limited field of view because of inevitable spin saturation and incomplete background suppression associated with short-T1 tissues, such as fat, gadolinium, and methemoglobin.

2D TOF is used to acquire a series of sequential thin-slice images over a large area, such as the extremities, neck, and abdomen. Each slice behaves as an entry slice, so that vessel enhancement is maximum. A presaturation band is applied above or below the slice to eliminate signal from vessels flowing in the opposite direction. If the vessel is perpendicular to the slice, the technique ensures that the signal of the vessel moving through the thin slice is maintained owing to its lack of saturation. 2D TOF imaging lends itself readily to imaging of fairly straight vessels, such as the carotids and peripheral vessels (see Fig. 8-3).

The voxel volume tends to be larger in 2D TOF imaging than in 3D TOF, thus reducing resolution. In addition, 2D pulse sequences often require the minimum TE to be longer as a result of increased work by the gradient in the acquisition of thin slices.

3D TOF imaging volumetrically acquires contiguous thin slices by the usual 3DFT method. 3D TOF imaging is the method of choice for imaging fast-flowing blood that does not particularly follow a straight course, such as the area surrounding the circle of Willis (see Fig. 8-4). The TE times tend to be shorter than with the 2D TOF

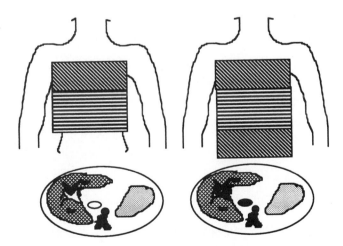

Figure 8-2   Effect of presaturation band placement on signal from blood.

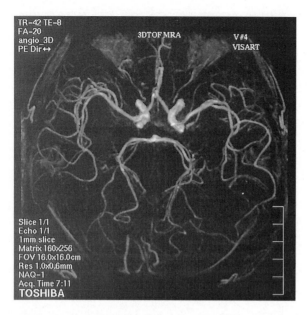

Figure 8-4 Vessels associated with the circle of Willis are nicely demonstrated using 3D TOF imaging with slice-selective off-resonance sinc (SORS) pulse presaturation. (*Courtesy Toshiba America Medical Systems, Inc. By permission.*)

method, resulting in minimized flow-turbulence-related artifacts. In addition, high-resolution images can be acquired, making the technique easily applicable to high-resolution MIP images. When voxel volumes are isotropic or nearly so, multiplanar reconstruction techniques used

to obtain images from the acquired data set produce images of high quality.

Table 8-2 compares 2D TOF vascular imaging with 3D TOF with regard to image quality and scan time.

Background Subtraction Technique—Phase-Shift Imaging

Phase-shift imaging (PSI), also called *phase contrast* (PC), differs from TOF in a very fundamental way: PSI techniques use velocity-induced phase shifts to differentiate moving spins from stationary spins. The contrast between flowing blood and stationary spins is related to blood velocity, so that a phase-difference image can be generated in which the blood vessel(s) will be bright and background tissue will have a cancellation effect.

In all forms of phase-shift imaging, *bipolar gradient pulses* are applied by velocity-encoding gradients. These consist of two lobes that are equal in amplitude and duration, but of opposite sign (+/−). The bipolar gradient pulses can be applied in one axis or in all three axes and

TABLE 8-2 2D TOF VERSUS 3D TOF VASCULAR IMAGING

	2DFT	3DFT
Clinical application	Slow flow, veins or arteries; abdominal vessels, extremities, carotid bifurcation—stenosis and occlusion, venous angiomas, basilar artery, intracranial venous thrombosis	Moderate to fast flow; intracranial arteries; carotid siphon, renal arteries, AVM nidus, aneurysm evaluation
Scan time	Very short; compatible with breath-hold techniques. Scan time based on 1 slice/TR. Total time dependent on coverage required	Long; dependent on 3D slice selection
Background suppression	Superior to 3D, but short-T1 tissue signal can simulate vascular enhancement	Short-T1 tissue may simulate vessel enhancement, causing incomplete background suppression
Resolution	Less than 3D because of slice thickness limitation; partial volume effects resulting from thickness of slice	High
SNR	Less than 3D; increased TE results in more T2 dephasing	High
Number of slices	Unlimited	Limited by scan time and inevitable spin saturation with increased volume traversed
FOV	Unlimited	Limited by inevitable spin saturation with increased volume traversed
MIP images	Increase in slice thickness may result in MIP artifacts	High resolution
Disadvantages	Lower SNR, decreased resolution, MIP artifacts (signal misregistration), poor sensitivity to in-plane flow	Insensitive to slow flow, limited FOV, incomplete background suppression, MIP artifacts

can be varied or chosen to depict fast, slow, or turbulent blood flow, depending on the clinical indication and the velocity-encoding value chosen.

Velocity-encoding gradients are used to generate similar waveforms for both acquisitions, but the direction of the waveform is reversed, resulting in a zero net area under the gradient waveform curve. Two sets of data are acquired, in which there is an alteration in the magnetic field gradient's strength and polarity. Because of this, stationary tissues do not accumulate a phase shift for either acquisition. However, moving spins will have accumulated a phase shift that is equal in magnitude but opposite in direction for the two acquisitions. This net accumulation is proportional to the flow velocity and the strength of the velocity-encoding gradient. The difference will result, after subtraction, in an image in which stationary tissue has no signal, while the signal of flowing blood is intense.

In the phase-shift method, a mask image is acquired with no flow sensitization, i.e., no bipolar gradient pulse. Successive images are acquired with the addition of specific strengths of bipolar gradients. The phase information from the encoded data sets is combined, and the mask data are subtracted away. Stationary tissue that is not affected by the bipolar pulses is eliminated from the resultant data set, leaving only the blood flow information. Net signal results after vector subtraction to obtain the difference image. This signal is roughly proportional to the sine of the phase difference. However, because of the cyclical nature of the sine function, a phase shift of 450° can appear the same as a phase shift of 90°, so that rapid flow produces the same signal as slow flow.[3] This is known as *aliasing* and can be avoided by reducing the strength of the flow-encoding gradient.

Gradient strength is specified as VENC (velocity-encoding), the minimum velocity at which aliasing will occur. If the approximate velocity of the vessel under examination is known, not only will the phenomenon of aliasing be avoided, but the vessel will be depicted much more accurately. By changing the amplitude of the flow-encoding pulse, it is possible to selectively generate an angiogram for a desired flow velocity (see Fig. 8-5). This indicates the spin speed which generates a phase change of one radian when the flow-encoding pulse is applied. A phase change of one radian is equal to π or 180°, which is the maximum phase shift possible. In other words, blood flow having a velocity component that is the same as the number of flow-encoding steps will have maximal enhancement.

The velocity of blood flow is defined by the distance traveled between the positive and negative lobes of the velocity-encoding gradient (a 180° phase shift will produce maximum signal intensity). It is given in centimeters per second. Table 8-3 gives peak velocities in adults. The VENC value chosen will cause the blood flow traveling at exactly that value in the direction of the positive lobe to be assigned the maximum pixel value. Blood flow in the opposite direction will be dark. Choose a VENC value

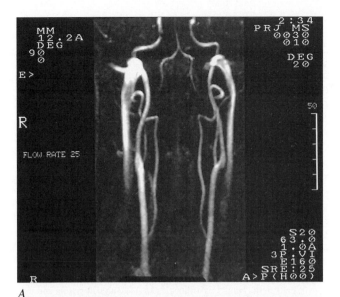

A

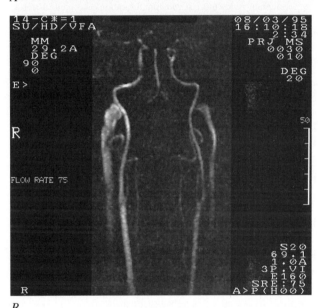

B

Figure 8-5 *A* and *B*. Phase-shift images using different velocity-encoding values. Note the aliasing artifacts with PSI using a flow rate of 25 cm/s; the image appears "splotchy" although the vascular signal is high.

slightly higher than the predicted velocity of the blood being observed to reduce the possibility of aliasing.

The velocity-encoding gradient can be applied in all three axes, depending on the direction and the blood flow velocity of the vessels being imaged. However, this technique is sensitive to flow only in the direction of the applied flow-encoding gradient. In cases of straight or relatively straight vessel orientation, such as the carotid arteries, this poses little problem, because they will add vectorially. However, in areas where there is multidirectional flow, as in the brain, the flow-encoding gradient must be applied in two or three orthogonal planes to produce the most accurate depiction of the vascular struc-

TABLE 8-3 PEAK BLOOD FLOW VELOCITIES IN ADULTS[a]

Vessels	Normal Peak Velocities	
Cerebral arteries	42–62 cm/s	+/− 11 cm/s
Carotid siphon	55 cm/s	+/− 13 cm/s
Basilar artery	40 cm/s	+/− 10 cm/s
Carotid arteries	80–120 cm/s	
Vertebral arteries	35 cm/s	+/− 9 cm/s
Aorta	100–175 cm/s	
External iliac	120 cm/s	+/− 21 cm/s
Superficial femorals	90 cm/s	+/− 14 cm/s
Popliteal	70 cm/s	+/− 13 cm/s
Common femoral	115 cm/s	
Veins	20 cm/s	

[a]Peak velocities for peripheral arteries were measured by duplex scanning; transcranial doppler measurements were obtained of arterial flow velocity in the head. Peak velocities are measured at systole and will vary considerably with exercise, anatomic location, and clinical status; systole drops off rapidly, so that the velocity of flow may decrease significantly during the cardiac cycle. [Adapted from Jager, Ricketts, Strandness, Jr.: Duplex scanning for the evaluation of lower limb arterial disease, in Berstein EF: *Non-Invasive Diagnostic Techniques in Vascular Disease,* St. Louis: Mosby, 1985, and Dewitt and Wechsler, *Stroke* 19(7), 1988.]

ture. Scan times can be considerable when more than one direction of encoding is specified, since two data sets are acquired for each encoding direction. Acquisition schemes are available that calculate data based on the accumulation of data sets in a single dimension by interpolating the negative node of the bipolar gradient from the acquired positive node, since both have the same amplitude. In any case, phase-shift imaging results in a longer scan time than do TOF techniques. In addition, since more data sets are acquired in which sophisticated mathematical calculations are performed, reconstruction time can be quite long and computer disk space usage is significant.

Phase-shift imaging can be performed using 2DFT or 3DFT methods, each of which has the same advantages and disadvantages encountered in general imaging. The 2D method can be used to produce multiple images, with the objective being speed of acquisition. This method has a number of advantages over the more time-consuming 3D schemes. It is most often done using slice thicknesses between 2 and 20 centimeters in which added coverage is required, such as when peripheral imaging of vessels is desired. When multidirectional flow-encoding gradients are necessary, 2D PSI techniques can be used to maintain shorter scan times. The direction of flow can be documented, and quantitative analysis of flow rates done, using 2D PSI as an addition to the more highly resolved 3D methods. Cardiac-gated PSI can be performed, where TR remains constant and each phase-encoding step is instituted by ECG triggering. Each phase of the cardiac cycle can be seen on the phase images because signal intensity is proportional to velocity and only one phase per slice is

being obtained for each repetition. Finally, 2D PSI can be used as a means of selecting the most appropriate VENC value for the vessel being imaged. By performing a very quick 2D sequence (less than 20-s scan time), different VENC values can be evaluated for use with the longer 3D PSI sequences.

2D PSI is used primarily as an adjunct to high-resolution vascular sequences such as 3D TOF or 3D PSI. It can be used in any anatomic region. In cases in which 3D imaging is not an option because of the slow velocity of blood flow in the region of interest, a series of thin 2D TOF slices through the area is suggested. A review of the 2D TOF MIP images that can be rotated may provide additional information.

3D PSI is highly effective at removing background signal. Therefore, enhancement of the vasculature can be documented for veins as well as arteries. In addition, with 3D technology, high-resolution images can be obtained in reasonable scan times.

Table 8-4 compares 2D and 3D PSI vascular imaging.

Practical Imaging Techniques

Vascular enhancement using magnetic resonance imaging can be optimized by following simple guidelines that tend to be common to all MRI techniques. That is, signal-to-noise ratio, contrast, and spatial resolution requirements are met by using techniques already established in MRI (see Part I). Current technology, such as presaturation and flow compensation, is used to maximize image quality on MR vascular scans by canceling the signal from background tissue as much as possible, allowing signal enhancement to be at its best. The use of magnetization transfer methods in 3D TOF imaging, discussed in Chap. 9, is one of these techniques.

Magnetization transfer contrast, or MTC, refers to a novel way of achieving contrast in MR images by using a radio-frequency preparation pulse that is similar to that used in inversion recovery (IR) imaging techniques, or by using an off-resonance RF pulse. It is a presaturation technique that helps to reduce the signal intensity from parenchyma, maximizing enhancement of vascular structures, especially in the peripheral vessels. This mechanism has been shown to improve flow contrast in the brain, because the bound pool (macromolecules in tissues) found in brain tissue has achieved a high rate of saturation. Other tissues that have high plasma membrane content, such as the kidney and muscle, also exhibit a significant degree of saturation transfer (see Table 8-5).

TABLE 8-4 2D PSI VERSUS 3D PSI VASCULAR IMAGING

	2DFT	3DFT
Clinical application	Both can be used to assess the following: large aneurysm with slow flow; assessment of AVM, arterial occlusive disease, venous occlusions and malformations, portal vein and associated diseases, peripheral vessels. 2D used as a prescan search for velocity-encoding gradient strength prior to lengthy 3D counterpart; 3D used for large-volume imaging	
Scan time	Very short; compatible with breath-hold techniques. Scan time based on 1 slice/TR. Total time dependent on coverage required	Long; dependent on 3D slice selection
Background suppression	Superior to 3D	High—free from problems related to short-T1 tissues
Resolution	Less than 3D because of slice thickness limitation; partial volume effects resulting from thickness of slice and phase dispersion	High—reduced phase dispersion effects
SNR	Less than 3D; minimum TE increased—more T2 dephasing	Higher than 2D; minimum TE increased to allow velocity encoding
Number of slices	Unlimited	Limited by scan time
FOV	Unlimited	Unlimited
MIP images	Increase in slice thickness may result in MIP artifacts	High resolution
Velocity encoding	Variable	Variable
Disadvantages	Eddy currents, one slice/data set—requires multiacquisition for multiple slices, intravoxel phase dispersion, high sensitivity to motion, susceptible to turbulence and pulsatility	Long scan time, eddy currents, intravoxel phase dispersion, high sensitivity to motion, susceptible to turbulence and pulsatility
	Multiacquisition required for multidirectional flow in both 2D and 3D imaging.	

Magnetization transfer techniques are generally spatially nonselective, so that the signal from inflowing blood can also become saturated. In order to improve the contrast between background tissue and inflowing blood, the effect MTC has on blood must be minimized. The use of MTC can be further optimized by using a slice-selective off-resonance sinc pulse (SORS).[4]

The SORS technique is essentially a selective presaturation technique that uses a slice gradient capable of maintaining the saturation pulse fairly close to the imaging volume (see Fig. 8-6). The critical factors in maximizing the effectiveness of the SORS presaturation band are the gradient strength and the ability of the Δf ("delta f," or change in frequency) to remain within a 5-kHz offset from the imaging volume. This is generally controlled via the design of the sinc pulse, which ideally has a very good slice profile. The advantages of the SORS technique are its selective magnetization transfer effect on background tissue, eliminating the signal from the venous sinus structures, and RF component adaptability.[5]

The choice of *scan parameters* in vascular studies using MRI is critical in producing images with the best vessel-to-background-tissue contrast. Table 8-6 provides helpful hints and explanations concerning selections of specific scan parameters. Other suggestions include:

1. Increase the TR to accommodate slower flow rates, such as those seen in some elderly patients.

TABLE 8-5 CONTRAST DIFFERENTIATION IN TISSUES WHERE MTC HAS BEEN USED

Saturated	Not Saturated	Contrast
Spinal cord	CSF	High
Cartilage	Synovial fluid	High
Brain tissue	In-flowing blood	High
Muscle	Fat	High

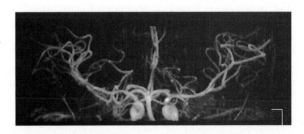

Figure 8-6 MR vascular image of brain using SORS technique. (*Courtesy Toshiba America Medical Systems, Inc. By permission.*)

TABLE 8-6 HELPFUL HINTS FOR VASCULAR IMAGING

Scan Parameter	Helpful Hints and Explanations
TE	Keep as short as possible to reduce dephasing effects. Minimum TE increases with use of flow compensation or in PSI imaging because of gradient requirements.
TR	Saturation effect of vessel can be reduced by increasing TR; however, scan time increases. Control vessel saturation using reduced FA. Background tissue saturation increases with decreased TR.
FA	A decrease in FA reduces saturation of flowing spins, thus improving signal.
FOV	Keep as small as possible to reduce intravoxel dephasing. Adjust phase- and frequency-encoding steps so that pixel size is fairly small (1 mm or so).
Slice thickness	Thin-slice imaging is necessary when imaging blood vessels. The slab thickness in 3D methods should be approximately the size of the vessel segment being imaged, generally 3 to 5 cm. In general, the thicker the slice, the greater the intravoxel dephasing, resulting in loss of signal.
N_{acq}	One acquisition is used in PSI for two reasons: There is no guarantee that the velocity of flow will be the same for additional passes of data collection, increasing the possibility for aliasing, and scan times increase proportionately.

2. Selective presaturation bands with 3D TOF imaging may not completely eliminate signal from spins within the saturation band. This can occur if the scanning region is parallel to the blood vessels, if the blood flow recovers from the saturation too quickly, or if paramagnetic agents such as gadolinium are added.
3. Signal loss in vessels may be observed in TOF imaging as a result of such phenomena as tortuosity of a vessel, susceptibility effects as they pass through the petrous ridges, or scan parameter selection that allows saturation of spins as they move through the slice or volume.
4. Coil selection is based on the need to optimize SNR for the body part being imaged. It is not likely that any surface coil will provide enough SNR to adequately visualize the vessels. Choose the coil that most closely corresponds in size to the region to be scanned.

Slice (2D) or *slab* (3D) orientation relative to vessel flow is paramount in producing images that depict the vessel adequately to allow evaluation. Vessels traverse the brain at varying angles. The choice of 2D versus 3D TOF

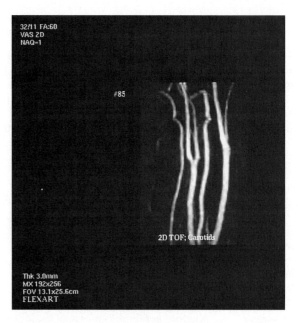

Figure 8-7 2D TOF vascular image of carotids.

imaging is usually dependent on the geometry of the vessel: is it straight or tortuous?

When performing 2D TOF, a locator sequence should be used to produce an image for scan planning. In 2D TOF imaging, the greatest time-of-flight effect occurs when flow is perpendicular to the slice plane (see Fig. 8-7). For this reason, the vascular images will usually be acquired in the axial plane, so your choice of locator plane should be one which allows you to plan an axial acquisition.

2D TOF imaging of the neck is generally performed to access the carotid bifurcation or upper neck vessels. The patient should be positioned more inferiorly in the coil to allow appropriate centering of the carotid bifurcation, which is approximately at the angle of the mandible (see Fig. 8-8). For general vascular imaging in the neck,

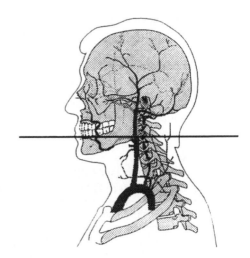

Figure 8-8 Centering for carotid bifurcation.

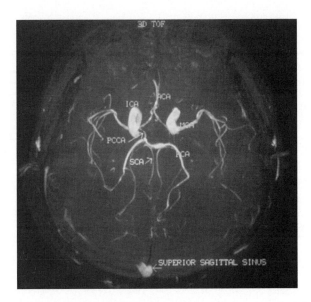

Figure 8-9   Circle of Willis using 3D TOF. (*Courtesy Toshiba America Medical Systems, Inc. By permission.*)

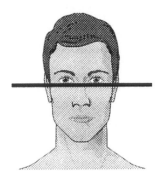

Figure 8-10   Infraorbital margin.

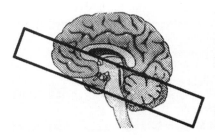

Figure 8-11   Positioning for circle of Willis. Alternative method: parallel with Reid's baseline.

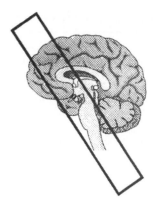

Figure 8-12   Positioning for basilar vessels.

positioning can be similar to that for general imaging of the cervical spine.

3D TOF and PSI techniques will most often be used for evaluating the intracranial vessels (see Fig. 8-9). Centering at or about the infra-orbital margin (Fig. 8-10), with the long axis of the body straight along the axis of the bore, is preferred by most investigators.

To visualize the anterior and posterior cerebral arteries and basilar artery, center the slab so that the inferior edge of the slab is about 1 cm below the pituitary. A true axial plane is preferred; this can be achieved by orienting the slab parallel to Reid's baseline. This is similar to the plane used in CT scanning (see Fig. 8-11).

A para-coronal plane is most often used to visualize the anterior cerebral artery, middle cerebral artery, basilar artery, upper internal carotid artery, and upper vertebral artery. Angle the slab so that it is parallel to the posterior surface of the clivus (see Figs. 8-12 and 8-13).

MR vascular imaging techniques have improved tremendously in the past five years. As knowledge about this technology continues to lead to increases in its reliability, questions about efficacy are replaced with accep-

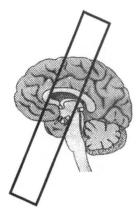

Figure 8-13   Positioning of middle cerebral artery along sylvian fissure.

TABLE 8-7 CLINICAL IMAGING GUIDELINES

Condition	Action	Effects on Image Quality
TR	Decrease TR	Improves suppression of stationary tissue.
		Decreases scan time.
	Increase TR	Improves time-of-flight effect; less spin saturation.
		Increases scan time.
TE	Decrease TE	Reduces flow-related dephasing from turbulence.
		Reduces effects of pulsatile flow motion.
		Minimum TE increases with flow compensation and PSI.
FA	Decrease FA	Improves time-of-flight effect.
	Increase FA	If TR is increased, provides adequate suppression of stationary tissue.
Slice or slab size	Decrease slice/slab thickness	Decreases intravoxel dephasing.
		Improves time-of-flight effect.
		Improves in-plane saturation in 2D TOF.
		Decreases scan time.
N_{acq}	Decrease N_{acq}	Decreases scan time.
		Decreases signal misregistration.
Slice/slab spacing	Increase shift	Decreases stepped-edge appearance.
		Decreases coverage.
MX	Increase matrix	Decreases partial volume effect.
		Decreases intravoxel dephasing.
FOV	Decrease FOV	Increases spatial resolution.
		Decreases intravoxel dephasing.
Saturation	Requires TR increase, FA decrease, and/or presaturation.	Eliminates flow-related enhancement from specific vessels (arterial versus venous).

TABLE 8-8 QUICK REFERENCE GUIDE TO IMPROVING VASCULAR ENHANCEMENT

Scan Parameter	Action	Effect
TR	Long	Less RF saturation
TE	Short	Less T2 dephasing
FA	Decrease	Less RF saturation
FC	Use of	Compensates for phase dispersion
Presat	MTC/SORS	Saturates stationary tissues
	Selective	Saturates opposing flow
FOV	Small	Reduces intravoxel dephasing
Slice	Small	Reduces intravoxel dephasing

sequence is performed and shows an apparent stenotic vessel. Since we know that time-of-flight methods can sometimes produce images with loss of signal at edges of the imaging volume, a subsequent 3D PSI sequence, which is not based on inflow enhancement, can be performed. If the result is similar to the observation obtained on the TOF image, confidence in the diagnosis is improved.

Table 8-7 identifies the effects that changes in scan parameters have on image quality. Table 8-8 provides a quick reference guide to methods of improving vascular enhancement.

References

1. Hylton NM, Winkler M, Du LN: Magnetic resonance angiography. *Diagnostic Imaging,* June 1990, pp 117–125.
2. Lee RE: MR angiographic imaging theory for the technologist, in Woodward P, Freimarck R: *MRI for Technologists.* New York: McGraw-Hill, 1995.
3. Borrello JS, Hylton NM, Du LN, Winkler M: Principles of magnetic resonance imaging, in Lanzer P, Yoganathar AP (eds): *Vascular Imaging by Color Doppler and Magnetic Resonance.* Springer-Verlag, 1991.
4. Miyazaki M et al.: A novel saturation contrast method for 3D time-of-flight magnetic resonance angiography: A slice-selective off-resonance sinc pulse (SORS) technique, *MRM* 32:52–58, 1994.
5. Miyazaki M et al.: A novel saturation contrast method for 3D time-of-flight magnetic resonance angiography: A slice-selective off-resonance sinc pulse (SORS) technique, MRM 32:52–58, 1994.

tance. By knowing the advantages and disadvantages of each MR vascular technique and applying that knowledge to the selection of the appropriate sequence and parameters, image optimization can be obtained.

In conclusion, MR vascular sequences are not unlike other MRI sequences. That is, if an area of question is discovered, evaluate the area further using different methods of vascular imaging. As an example, a 3D TOF

Suggested Readings

Elster AD: *Questions and Answers in Magnetic Resonance Imaging*. St. Louis: Mosby, 1994.

Iwamoto K, Fukushima M, Futami H: Usefulness of saturation transfer contrast in cerebral magnetic resonance angiography, *Medical Review* 49:20–24.

9 Magnetization Transfer Imaging

The human body is made up of both solid and liquid material, with the bulk of the liquid being water. Current clinical MR imaging is based primarily upon signals that are emitted from protons found in freely moving water molecules. One of the basic concepts of MR imaging is that water molecules emit MR signals that possess a long T2. The T2 for these freely moving water molecules is generally on the order of multiples of tens of milliseconds.

In addition to these freely moving water molecules, there are also protons that are less freely moving; these are typically found in more solid structures of the body. They are commonly referred to as proteins and hydrated water molecules, and typically possess T2s of less than 1 ms. MRI is relatively "blind" to these molecules, since they are not directly visible in routine clinical MR imaging as a result of their very short T2. However, these relatively immobile protons influence the relaxation times of the more freely moving protons used for MR imaging.

Magnetization transfer (MT) techniques provide information regarding the interaction that occurs between the relatively fixed and the relatively free moving protons found in the human body. MT allows for the measurement of the exchange rate of magnetization between these two types of protons, and as a result represents a type of MR contrast. MT MR contrast can be generated by using specific MR techniques. These involve applying RF pulses that affect both the relatively free protons (Hf) and the more restricted protons (Hr). For example, in the formation of MT MR contrast, Hr can be saturated with an off-resonance RF pulse (one that does not affect Hf). However, because the magnetization of Hr interacts with that of Hf, Hr magnetization is transferred to Hf. This interaction decreases the amount of signal emitted by Hf.

The amount of the saturation transferred depends on several factors, including the size of the Hr molecule, the efficiency of the exchange rate between Hf and Hr, and the amplitude, duration, and frequency of the applied off-resonance RF pulse (Figs. 9-1 and 9-2).

MT MR contrast enables improved visualization of both lipid-containing and water-containing structures. This is because the magnetization of protons found in mobile lipid molecules is not affected by the off-resonance RF pulse that is applied during the use of MT. These protons of mobile lipid molecules simply do not interact with Hr as do the Hf molecules. Therefore, the signal from the lipid molecules is not decreased when Hr magnetization is transferred to Hf. This interaction decreases the amount of signal emitted by Hf but not the amount of signal emitted by the lipid (fatty) structures.

Likewise, there is less magnetization transfer to Hf from an off-resonance RF pulse in structures with a very high water content. Therefore, the signal from the high-water-content lesions is not decreased when Hr magnetization is transferred to Hf, since there is less protein in these structures. This interaction decreases the amount of signal emitted by Hf in normal tissues, but not the amount of signal emitted by these higher-water-content lesions.

In addition to improving the visualization of abnormalities with high lipid and water content, MT has been shown to improve the effect of paramagnetic contrast agents. Basically, the MT contrast decreases the signal from normal tissue, but does not affect the signal from paramagnetic contrast agents. In the same manner in which MT works for lipid- and high-water-containing structures, it is effective for lesions containing paramagnetic contrast. The MT process is relatively specific to the

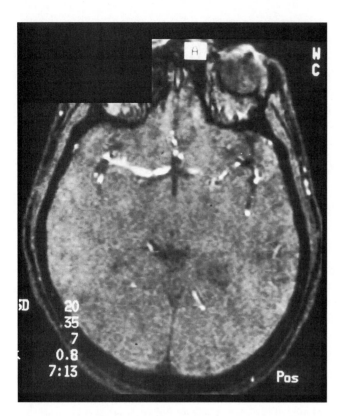

Figure 9-1　Axial GRE MR (TR 35, TE 7, FA 20) performed for MRA without magnetization transfer, demonstrating increased signal from intracranial vessels with suppression of background brain signal. (Compare to Fig. 9-2.)

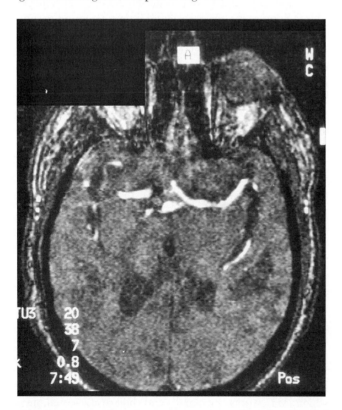

Figure 9-2　Axial GRE MR (TR 38, TE 7, FA 20) performed for MRA with magnetization transfer, demonstrating increased signal from intracranial vessels with improved suppression of background brain signal. (Compare to Fig. 9-1.)

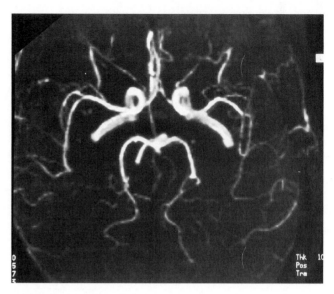

Figure 9-3　Magnetic resonance angiography maximum intensity projection performed without magnetization transfer. (Compare to Fig. 9-4.)

interactions of water and macromolecules, so that the interactions of protons and paramagnetic contrast agents are minimally affected. Therefore, protons interacting with paramagnetics do not interact with Hr as do the Hf molecules. The signal from the paramagnetic effect is not decreased when Hr magnetization is transferred to Hf. This interaction decreases the amount of signal emitted by Hf in the normal tissues, but not the amount of signal emitted by the paramagnetic-containing structures. This reduction in background (normal tissue) signal in effect increases the amount of signal from the paramagnetically enhanced lesions. This could be referred to as MT contrast enhancement of an MR contrast-enhanced lesion.

MT can be applied to any method that benefits from

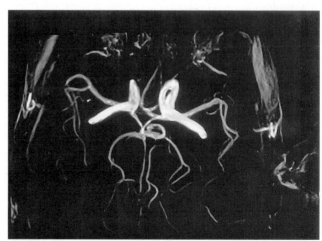

Figure 9-4　Magnetic resonance angiography maximum intensity projection performed with magnetization transfer. (Compare to Fig. 9-3 and note the improved definition of the intracranial vasculature.)

a reduction in the amount of signal emitted from normal tissue. Therefore, in addition to lipids, high-water-content structures, and paramagnetically enhanced lesions, MT can be applied to magnetic resonance angiography (MRA). In this technique, MT is performed as an added method of tissue subtraction, with a resulting increase in signal from flowing blood. The gray matter of the brain and saturated blood have a similar signal. Therefore, the application of an MT sequence that suppresses both the gray and white matter will result in a consequent increase in vessel visualization (see Figs. 9-1 and 9-2). The better the background brain tissue is suppressed, the better the visualization of small intracranial vessels as well as the lu-men of larger vessels (Figs. 9-3 and 9-4). This is one of the more common uses of MT in routine clinical practice.

Suggested Readings

Stark DD, Bradley WG Jr: *Magnetic Resonance Imaging.* St. Louis, MO: Mosby-Year Book, 1986.

10

Fat-Suppression Techniques

Clinical MR imaging consists of signal identification of the hydrogen atoms in tissues. Most of the hydrogen is contained in water and lipid components, both of which can be readily seen on MRI. T1 and T2 relaxation characteristics for simple water- and fat-containing structures are well known (see Fig. 10-1). Generally, fat is seen as a bright signal on conventional T1-weighted images and as less bright on T2-weighted images. However, it can be very bright on fast spin echo T2-weighted images as well, because of the T1 contributions of early sampled echoes (see Chap. 7). Generally, fluid-filled structures are dark on T1- and bright on T2-weighted images.

Structures containing significant amounts of free hydrogen, as is found in most simple fluids, are in well-organized compartments of the body, such as the urinary bladder, ventricular system, and ocular bulb. Fat surrounds many of these structures but is not as well circumscribed. In some tissues, fat is a molecular component along with hydrogen in fluids. Increased hydrogen concentration as it relates to disease processes is the hallmark of abnormal versus normal tissues as they appear using MRI. The most common example is found in diseased fatty bone marrow, where an increased amount of hydrogen protons is found in the fatty marrow and is due to the inflammatory response of the body to the pathology. Many times it is difficult to separate the fat from water, so that diagnostic ability is hampered.

Clinically, fat-suppression techniques in the form of gradient echo out-of-phase imaging, STIR, and Dixon techniques have been employed for many years. However, there is often lack of uniformity of suppression, especially when imaging large fields of view, such as the chest and abdomen, that have a wide range of frequencies. As a result, several MR imaging techniques have been devel-

oped that are much more sophisticated in suppressive abilities than their previous counterparts. This chapter is devoted to explanations of the procedures available, old and new, that help to differentiate fat from disease.

STIR

The simplest fat-suppression technique, STIR (short-TI inversion recovery), has been commonly used to reduce the signal from fat so that fluid-filled areas, such as diseased bone marrow, can be more readily identified. This technique is merely an inversion recovery sequence that uses a short TI time, usually in the range of 60 to 170 ms rather than the 400 to 600 ms of conventional IR imaging. The clinical advantages of STIR are based on its additive T1 and T2 contrast, significant fat-suppression capabilities, and a magnetization recovery range that is twice that of a spin echo sequence. This produces images with high lesion contrast and conspicuity.[1]

STIR imaging for fat suppression is based on the premise that when a tissue vector crosses the transverse plane after an inverting pulse of 180°, no appreciable signal can be obtained; it is insignificant or "nulled." The null point has been identified as the point at which the tissue vector is at or near the transverse plane. This is the halfway point between the positive Z and negative Z directions, and so collectively the longitudinal magnetiza-

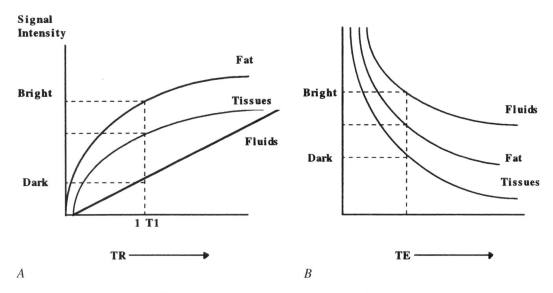

Figure 10-1   General T1 and T2 relaxation curves. A. T1 growth curve. B. T2 relaxation curve.

tion is zero. The null point has been determined to be approximately 69 percent of the T1 relaxation time of a tissue, making STIR a field-strength-dependent technique. As with any inversion recovery sequence, following the 180° RF inverting pulse, the tissue vectors proceed through recovery from the negative Z longitudinal axis, which has 100 percent magnetization, to the transverse plane, which has no longitudinal magnetization. In terms of signal appearance, the tissues recover from a point at which signal is maximum (-Z longitudinal magnetization) to one at which no signal is obtainable (transverse). Eventually, if TI time is long enough, the vectors will return to positive longitudinal magnetization and maximum signal intensity. The ability of the tissue to elicit a unique signal is dependent on both the TI time and the TR, which are chosen by the operator.

TI time is based on the T1 relaxation time of the tissue one wishes to suppress (see Fig. 10-2). When TI time is chosen to be at or close to the null point for that tissue, little or no signal will be available during subsequent data sampling. If fat suppression is the objective, all tissues which are composed of or surrounded by fat will show very little, if any, signal intensity. Since a good deal of the molecular structure of the human body contains some form of lipid material, and that material has been suppressed, the images have the appearance of being "signal-starved." However, the contrast between fat and fluid is remarkable (see Fig. 10-3).

The repetition time TR also has a profound effect on image contrast when inversion recovery imaging such as STIR is performed. It controls the amount of time allowed for longitudinal recovery (albeit from the negative direction to the positive direction) before data sampling is initiated. Therefore, if the objective is to observe a signal void from fat along with a bright signal from CSF, TR

must be adequately high, much like that used for T2-weighted imaging. However, the time component of STIR sequences then tends to be high, resulting in more flow and motion artifacts.

When attempting to suppress the signal from fat, one must realize that there are variations in the type of fat and the molecular structure of fat in tissues that may have an effect on the suppression of the signal. For example, retro-orbital fat, which is not tightly bonded with other tissues, may be suppressed more than fat contained in bony trabecula. What this means is that a TI time that may suppress fat well when used for optic nerve imaging may not be as effective when imaging for bone marrow. Targeting the TI specifically to the anatomic region will produce the best overall suppression of fat signal.

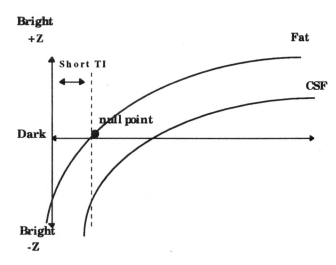

Figure 10-2   TI selection relative to tissue signal intensity using 180° inverting pulse of IR sequence.

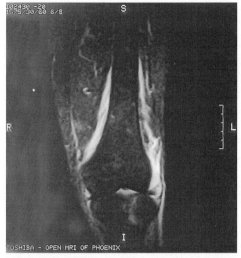

A

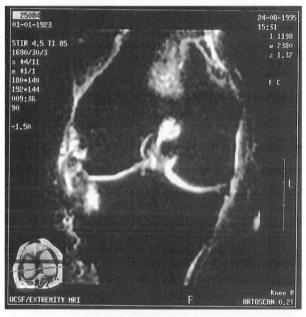

B

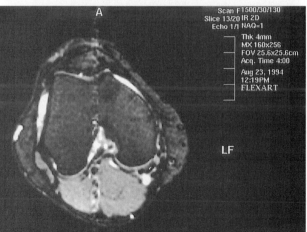

C

Figure 10-3 TI is field-strength-dependent. STIR images as seen using field strength of 0.064 T *(A) (courtesy Open MRI of Phoenix; by permission)*, 0.2 T *(B) (courtesy LUNAR Corporation; by permission)*, and 0.5 T *(C)*.

Inversion recovery imaging, like any sequence, requires optimum tuning by manufacturer service personnel to ensure that the flip angles are accurate for the pulse sequence design. If the flip angle is actually 150° rather than 180°, for example, spins will recover as usual, but pass the null point, where signal would be zero. Subsequent flip angles (90° and 180° refocusing) will be askew as well. If fat suppression is the objective, it will not be optimized, as the fat-tissue vector will already have crossed the null point on its way to positive longitudinal magnetization. The fat will therefore appear gray, and so fat suppression will not have been accomplished. This can have an effect on other tissues as well. If the CSF vector is recovering from 150°, at the time the data are sampled it will be in the gray zone of negative longitudinal recovery instead of in the bright zone (see Fig. 10-2). If the apparent signal intensity is not as expected for the TI chosen, consider evaluation of the sequence tuning by service personnel.

STIR images have historically had a less desirable appearance than conventional images. They have high contrast and low signal, which makes them less pleasing. If the MR system is not well maintained or has problems with field homogeneity, images may appear even worse. Additionally, if good MR imaging techniques are not practiced, objects that have an effect on the magnetic field may interfere with the achievement of optimum image quality.

STIR imaging increases lesion detection and conspicuity, but is not necessarily considered a high-resolution technique. It is commonly used as an adjunct to the routine sequences used for the clinical indication. Since STIR images, by virtue of the physics of the sequence, contain less signal than conventional spin echo images, methods of generating more signal can be used. This can be accomplished by developing protocols that will improve the signal-to-noise ratio of the image at the expense of a slight loss in resolution. An increase in the slice thickness or a decrease in the number of matrix steps will increase the voxel volume, which will help to improve SNR. The lowest TE should be chosen to minimize T2 decay. TR should be high enough to allow for almost complete longitudinal recovery of all tissue vectors following data collection. Artifact-suppression techniques such as flow compensation, gating, or presaturation can be used to compensate for flow and respiratory motion. (However, in such areas as the lungs, which contain many blood vessels, flow compensation may not be clinically useful because of its effect on producing high signal in those vessels. Antialiasing techniques can be used to minimize loss of detail resulting from wraparound artifacts. It may be advantageous to acquire images using conjugate symmetry, such as half-Fourier imaging, so that more signal averaging can be employed to reduce artifacts without adversely affecting scan time. All in all, protocols using thicker slices, fewer encoding steps, larger fields of view, partial data set techniques, and more signal averaging can

TABLE 10-1 CLINICAL INDICATIONS FOR STIR

CNS	Bone	Soft Tissue
Demyelinating disease	Avascular necrosis	Popliteal cysts
Neoplasms	Marrow edema	Meniscal cysts
Optic neuritis	Marrow infarcts	Ganglions
Brachial plexus	Trabecular microfractures	Metastatic disease
	Effusions	Osteomyelitis
		Diskitis
		Intrasubstance tears of cruciate ligaments or patellar tendon
		Neoplasms
		Infections
		Intraabdominal or pelvic tumor involvement

Source: Adapted from Porter BA: *STIR* imaging—a technical review and current status, from Syllabus Material, Magnetic Resonance Imaging Conference (MRIC) for technologists, San Francisco, February 1993.

be employed to generate STIR images with fairly high SNR and fewer artifacts in a minimum of scan time. Table 10-1 identifies many of the clinical indications for performing a supplemental STIR sequence.

STIR imaging can be extremely useful in detecting and assessing lesions by adequately suppressing the signal from fat. When it is used as a supplemental sequence in routine imaging, confidence in its capability will increase with experience. It is a very easy imaging technique that when optimized for SNR can produce a high yield.

Chemical Shift Imaging

Chemical shift is a phenomenon in MR imaging that can produce an artifact that obscures fat/water boundaries. This occurs because of a shifted fat signal in the readout direction when a voxel contains both fat and water components. It is visible as a black line of several pixel widths

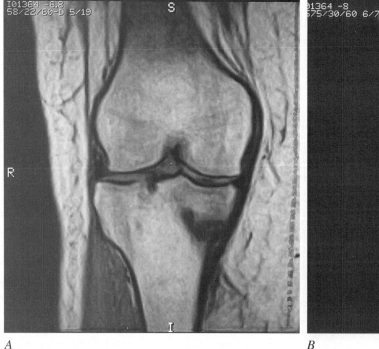
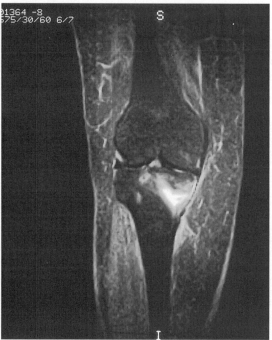

A *B*

Figure 10-4 Proton-density *(A)* and STIR *(B)* coronal images of knee. *(Courtesy Open MRI of Phoenix. By permission.)*

at the interface of fat and water and is a result of differences in the precessional frequency between fat and water. Fourier transform is not able to distinguish the frequency shift produced by chemical factors from the distribution frequencies produced by the readout gradient. The computer misinterprets this as a disparity in spatial location along the frequency-encoding direction. The displacement of fat-generated signal creates an artifactual gap or signal void at one edge of a tissue interface, which will be visible in the readout direction (see Fig. 10-5).

Chemical shift becomes worse with increasing field strength and narrow-bandwidth sequences (see Chap. 6). However, this phenomenon may be exploited to produce a form of fat suppression when using gradient echo or spin echo technology. Sometimes these techniques are referred to as "phase evolution" methods of fat suppression. In order to understand these techniques, it is necessary to understand the mechanism of chemical shift.

An atom has two main components: a nucleus, which contains at least one proton and, in all elements except H[1], at least one neutron, and one or more electron clouds that surround the atom. A consequence of the NMR experiment is the induction of electric currents in the electron cloud by exposure of a molecule to an external magnetic field. The electrons begin to circulate, generating a secondary magnetic field which weakens the local magnetic field experienced by the proton. This can be thought of as a form of electronic shielding at the atomic level (see Fig. 10-6). Additionally, the orbiting electrons can generate a magnetic field about neighboring nuclei that may either oppose or reinforce the proton's field.[2]

The amount of shielding experienced by the protons will depend on the molecular structure of the tissue or to what the atom is attached. For example, if the atom is attached to an electronegative atom, such as oxygen in water molecules, the shielding is relatively weak (see Fig. 10-7). This is because oxygen draws the electron cloud

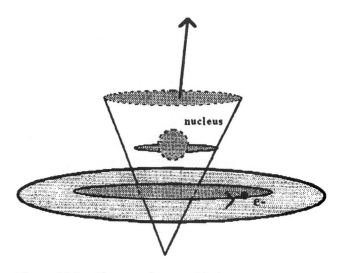

Figure 10-6 Electron orbit around hydrogen atom generates a secondary magnetic field which can shield the magnetic field of the nucleus.

away from the proton. If the shielding is weak, the proton within the nucleus maintains a stronger local magnetic field and a faster precessional frequency.

Hydrogen atoms in fat molecules are attached to carbon, which is less electronegative than oxygen. This results in stronger shielding of the hydrogen proton because of the closer proximity of the electron cloud to the nucleus. The stronger the shielding, the weaker the magnetism of the proton and the slower its precessional frequency. Therefore, fat molecules precess more slowly than water molecules (see Fig. 10-8).

The difference in precessional frequency between fat and water is known as chemical shift and is approximately 3.5 parts per million (ppm). Chemical shift is expressed in parts per million since this unit is independent of field

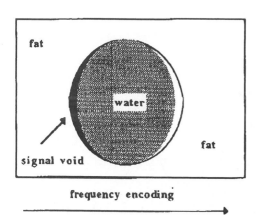

Figure 10-5 Illustration of chemical shift artifact depicting spatial misregistration of the fat versus water signal. If a fat molecule was residing in water, the bands of signal void and increased signal would be swapped.

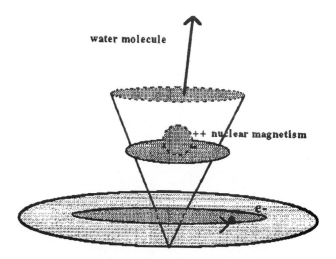

Figure 10-7 Water molecule exhibits strong nuclear magnetism and therefore higher precessional frequency because of the relative distance of the orbiting electron from the proton.

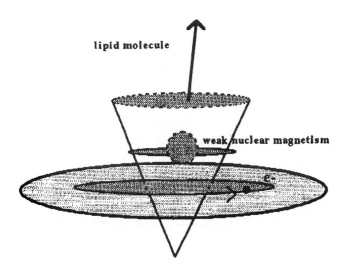

Figure 10-8   Lipid molecule exhibits weak nuclear magnetism and therefore lower precessional frequency as a result of the close proximity of the orbiting electron, which shields the proton from the externally applied magnetic field.

strength. The reference point that is used to measure chemical shifts is that of tetramethylsilane (TMS), because silicon has a low electronegativity. The shielding of protons in this compound is greater than in most other organic molecules, so that the NMR signals of most other molecules are shifted in the same direction downfield from TMS. TMS is assigned a frequency shift of 0.0 ppm; most other organic molecules have chemical shifts between 0 and 10 ppm.

Water has a chemical shift of 4.7 ppm, and most lipids have a chemical shift of 1.2 ppm; hence the 3.5-ppm difference (see Fig. 10-9). The frequency difference at various field strengths can be determined by multiplying the operating frequency of the MR system by 3.5 (see Table 10-2).

Actually, we want to know the chemical shift of certain elements because this is the basis of our ability to determine fat distribution within tissues. It helps us to distinguish a variety of liver and bone marrow diseases, such as liver degeneration by fatty infiltration, cirrhosis, hepatitis, and bone marrow necrosis. We thus exploit this phenomenon to create images that will be of use.

Fat-suppression chemical shift imaging uses pulse sequence designs to cancel the signal from fat. The simplest fat-suppression technique occurs as a result of fat and water tissues residing in the same voxel when using gradient echo imaging. The phenomenon is exploited by using an echo time that reduces the signal from fat because of phase cancellation of the fat/water spins at the time of data sample (see Fig. 10-10).

When fat and water are present in the same voxel, a chemical shift between them results in a spatial misregistration for several pixel widths. Following RF excitation, at TE = 0, both fat and water are in phase with respect to each other. Their signals are additive, so that at TE = 0, maximum signal intensity is achieved. When the signals are additive, the spins are said to be "in phase." As TE increases, the fat and water spins begin to precess at their characteristic frequency. Because of chemical shift, their signals will proceed through T2 decay at different rates and eventually move 180° out of phase with each other. When their phase relationship is exactly opposite, their signals will cancel and the signal intensity in the voxel will be minimal. With further increases in TE, fat and water will cycle in and out of phase with each other (see Fig. 10-11). The signal intensities will be brightest when in phase, and darkest when out of phase (see Fig. 10-12).

The contrast resulting from phase cycling can be used to effectively suppress the signal from fat when performing gradient echo imaging techniques.

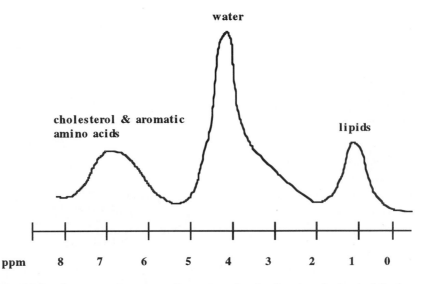

Figure 10-9   Spectroscopic pattern of organic molecules found at the level of the human liver.

TABLE 10-2 FREQUENCY DIFFERENCE BETWEEN FAT AND WATER AT VARIOUS FIELD STRENGHTS

Field Strength, T	Frequency Difference, Hz
0.064	9.5
0.2	30
0.35	52
0.5	75
1.0	149
1.5	224

If an echo time when the spins' phases are 180° out of phase is chosen, the signal for fat will be minimal. The degree to which fat suppression occurs is dependent on the amount and proportion of fat and water in a given voxel. If the ratio is 1:1, then complete cancellation will occur when the spins are out of phase. If the voxel contains only fat, then suppression will not occur because there has been no contribution from water signal.

The echo times relevant to in-phase/out-of-phase imaging are field-strength-dependent. They can be calculated from the frequency difference of the operating system (see Table 10-2). The formula takes the inverse of the difference and converts it to milliseconds:

1/frequency difference = TE (milliseconds)

For example, at an operating system of 1.5 tesla, the chemical shift frequency difference is 224 Hz, so that $1/224 = 0.00446$, or 4.5 ms. That means that every 4.5 ms, the phases of fat and water are cycling in and out of phase with each other. For images where the fat and water signals are additive and therefore maximum, choosing an echo time of TE = 4.5 ms will yield in-phase im-

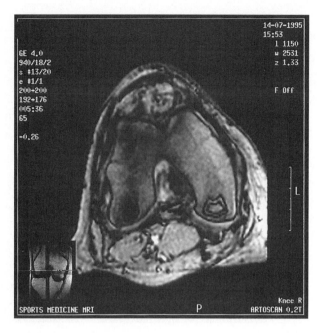

Figure 10-10 Out-of-phase gradient echo image of the knee. *(Courtesy LUNAR Corporation. By permission.)*

ages. Out-of-phase images, where the signal from fat has been suppressed, can be generated by selecting a TE that is approximately one-half the in-phase TE and adding it to the in-phase value. Multiples of both the in-phase and out-of-phase TE can be used to generate images. Table 10-3 charts these relationships for various field strengths.

Sample in-phase/out-of-phase calculations:

Field strength	1.0 tesla
Larmor frequency	42.58 MHz/T $\times$ 1.0 T = 42.58 MHz = 42.6 MHz

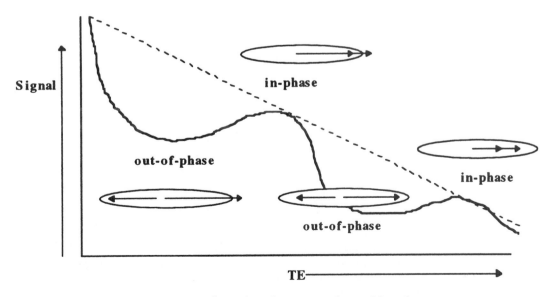

Figure 10-11 Relationship of TE to spin phases of fat and water.

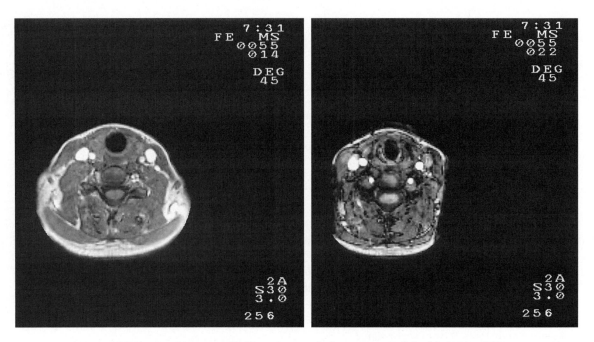

Figure 10-12   In-phase image (left) versus out-of-phase image (right) of the cervical spine.

Chemical shift   3.5 ppm × 42.6 MHz = 149.1 Hz
                  = 149 Hz
In-phase TE   1/149 = 0.0067 = 6.7 ms;
                  therefore 6.7,13.4, 20.1, . . .
Out-of-phase TE   6.7/2 = 3.35 = 3.4 ms; therefore
                  3.4 + 6.7 = 10.1, 16.8, 23.5 . . .

Out-of-phase chemical shift images appear as if a black line has been drawn about all fat/water interfaces. It is symmetric about the interfaces, as compared to the chemical shift artifact, in which one edge of the interface has a signal void while the opposite edge portrays as bright signal. The advantages of this type of fat suppression include superb edge enhancement of fat/water interfaces, a decrease in the signal from fat-containing structures, and a reduction in the chemical shift artifact and therefore the confusion arising from that artifact. Furthermore, an increase in the ability to characterize high-signal-intensity structures on T1-weighted images, such as differences be-

tween the increased signal normally associated with fat and that from hemorrhage (the fat signal is voided, whereas the signal from hemorrhage remains intense), is advantageous. The disadvantages include a slight decrease in the apparent size of pathology at the interface as a result of the size of the pixel shift (which increases with field strength and narrow-bandwidth imaging) and a decrease in SNR as a result of gradient echo technology. In addition, magnetic susceptibility increases when gradient echo imaging is performed, so that areas where this is more apparent, such as the region of the pituitary and the sphenoid and ethmoid sinuses, appear to have significant signal voids.

Another method that exploits the chemical shift phenomenon was developed by Dixon in 1984.[3] The scheme is a 2DFT hydrogen proton chemical shift technique that obtains images with excellent spatial resolution that can resolve the chemical shifts of two spectral lines, water and lipid (see Fig. 10-13).

In the original method, commonly referred to as the

TABLE 10-3 IN-PHASE AND OUT-OF-PHASE TE

Field Strength (T)	0.64	0.15	0.2	0.35	0.5	1.0	1.5	2.0
Frequency, MHz	2.73	6.4	8.5	15	21.3	42.6	63.9	85.2
Chemical shift, Hz	9.6	22.4	30	52.5	75	149	224	298
In-phase TE, ms	104	44.6	33.3	19.0	13.3	6.7	4.5	3.4
Out-of-phase TE, ms	52	22.3	16.7	9.5	6.7	3.4	2.3	1.7

Note: In-phase and out-of-phase echo times depicted are the calculated times of cycling. Multiples of these values are generally used as the TE that yields either an out-of-phase or in-phase image. Consult the operator's guide for the system you are using for exact TE values.

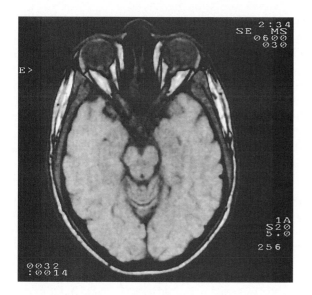

Figure 10-13   Dixon image of optic nerve.

ences but doesn't compensate for field inhomogeneities (see Fig. 10-14). Because gradient echo imaging is performed as a part of this sequence, the Dixon method of fat suppression suffers from the usual problems associated with gradient echo imaging, such as magnetic field inhomogeneities, motion, and susceptibility effects. However, it also results in the characteristic chemical shift effects seen in gradient echo imaging, the objective of performing the sequence. Reconstruction of the data sets therefore is complicated by additional factors (other than chemical shift) that affect the phase of the MR signal.

Variants of the Dixon technique were developed to bypass the usual scheme of double-set acquisition, thereby reducing scan time, and to compensate for factors that have plagued the method. Most, however, still require elaborate postprocessing methods and have been replaced by more sophisticated versions of fat suppression.

Dixon technique is performed, which is the acquisition of a pair of spin echo data sets, where one set uses a conventional 180° refocusing pulse to produce in-phase spins, while the other uses an offset version of the refocusing pulse to generate out-of-phase signals. When the reference point for the transmitter is set to the precessional frequency of water, addition and subtraction of the two data sets yields water- and fat-only images, respectively.[4] The amount of offset is determined by a time approximately equal to one-quarter the difference in frequency of the components being evaluated.[5]

The use of a conventional 180° refocusing pulse results in masking of differences in frequency between hydrogen-containing components and corrections for field inhomogeneities. However, the decentered 180° nature of the opposed phase echo employs a gradient reversal as well, which allows for expression of the phase-shift differ-

Advanced Fat-Suppression Techniques

Frequency-selective excitation or saturation sequences, such as "fat sat" and CHESS (chemical shift selection), use variations in the way the RF pulse is applied and when it is applied. In the pure sense of fat saturation, fat is selectively saturated by using a narrow-bandwidth frequency-selective prep pulse of long duration. This pulse effectively rotates the fat vector about the direction of the applied RF field while T1 and T2 relaxation are occurring so that the fat signal is driven to zero. A conventional pulse sequence is then used to obtain only the signal from

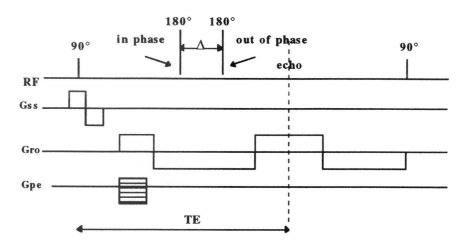

Figure 10-14   Dixon method using modified spin echo with gradient echo technique.

water. This method of fat suppression is time-consuming and requires high RF power, which increases patient SAR levels.

Fat signal can be "spoiled" by using gradients to cause dephasing of its spins. A variation of the method, *CHESS*, requires a short-duration frequency-selective 90° RF pulse to rotate the fat vector into the transverse plane, where spoiler gradients are used to force continued dephasing of the fat spins. Theoretically, only water's magnetization in the Z axis is available for signal production. However, difficulty arises in obtaining complete fat saturation without affecting water signal. This may be a result of nonpure RF sidebands that cause incomplete fat saturation and/or partial saturation of water components. Other problems associated with spectral selective imaging are related to T1 contrast seen in brain imaging, which appears different from that seen in conventional images.

Many versions of fat suppression have been developed that are outgrowths of the methodology previously described. Included is a version that acquires all the information necessary for separating water and fat signals in a single scan, using a *"sandwich" spin echo sequence* that is also capable of multiple-echo acquisition.[6] The technique was developed to compensate for difficulties in separating

fat and water arising from field inhomogeneities when using multiple RF pulses in the Dixon technique, especially at lower field strengths, where the frequency difference is small. Because of the longer time period necessary for the phase cycle at lower field strengths (see Table 10-3, out-of-phase TE), more k-space data can be acquired by collecting several field echoes before the 180° refocusing pulse. This method, as stated by Zhang et al., may be useful in separating multiple spectral lines, such as fat, water, and silicon.

Slice-selective gradient reversal techniques use a narrow-bandwidth 90° pulse in conjunction with a reduced strength in the slice select gradient. This induces an emphasized chemical shift misregistration in the slice direction. It is followed by a gradient reversal of the slice select gradient during the 180° refocusing pulse. Fat protons are shifted out of the slice plane and therefore do not receive both 90° and 180° pulses. That leaves only the water component, which has been stimulated by both, to produce signal.

Newer techniques, developed to suppress the signal from fat while preserving the gray/white T1 contrast in the brain, use *polarity-altered spectral and spatial selective acquisition* techniques (see Fig. 10-15). The tech-

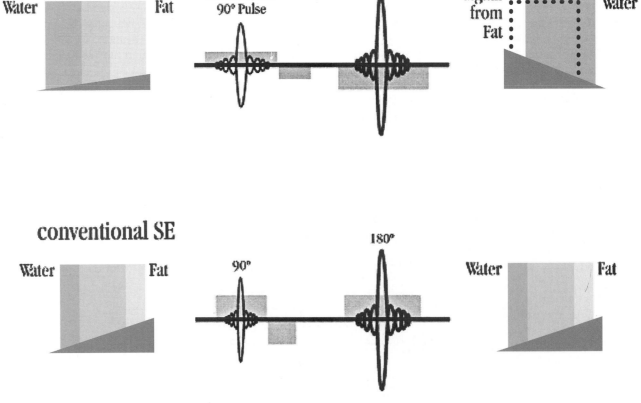

Figure 10-15 Graphic illustration of PASTA pulse sequence versus conventional pulse sequence. *(Courtesy Toshiba America Medical Systems, Inc. By permission.)*

nique, PASTA, uses a narrow-band spectral selective 90° pulse to eliminate fat signals and an altered polarity for 90° and 180° gradients to avoid contamination of fat signals.[7]

Unlike CHESS, the PASTA technique suppresses the signal from fat with no loss of water signal (see Fig. 10-16). The T1 contrast observed is compatible with that of conventional SE.

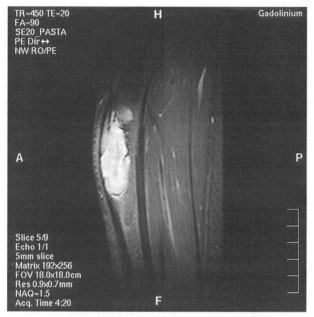

A

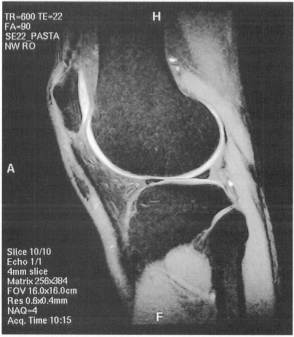

B

Figure 10-16 PASTA images of *(A)* the leg and *(B)* the knee. *(Courtesy Toshiba America Medical Systems, Inc. By permission.)*

Uniform fat suppression using the conventional methods described earlier in this chapter, especially when large fields of view, such as the chest, are imaged, is difficult to obtain because of the widely varying frequencies that are encountered in the tissues. High-order shims may resolve some of this problem but are not practical for clinical use. First-order shimming is effective; however, when the slice moves from the isocenter, the frequency is shifted in the readout direction. A fat-suppression method developed for multislice imaging uses an off-resonance pre-pulse for each slice. The sequence is called *MSOFT* (multislice off-resonance fat-suppression technique).[8]

Selective off-resonance fat saturation is accomplished using MSOFT by performing first-order shimming in the X, Y, and Z directions prior to acquisition. During this time, frequency-domain information for each slice is quickly sampled and recorded. A fat-suppression pulse that is specific to each frequency offset is preset and applied for each slice. When multislice imaging is performed over large areas such as the chest and abdomen, where large frequency shifts are common as a result of susceptibility effects, this scheme provides uniform fat suppression throughout the entire imaged volume (see Fig. 10-17). MSOFT also is beneficial when imaging smaller FOVs because of its precision in fat suppression.

New techniques for minimizing the exceedingly bright signal from fat on fast spin echo images have been developed. The high fat signal is a product of the contribution of lower echoes to the effective TE, which, depending on the echo-train length and echo-train spacing, can result in more T1 weighting. With smaller echo-train spacing, the signal from fat increases, which in many cases is undesirable. Methods such as low-bandwidth off-resonance RF pulse fat saturation are limited by field inhomogeneities and flip angle errors, often resulting in higher than expected fat signal.[9] In conventional fast spin echo imaging, the echoes are evenly spaced to synchronize with the phase of the stimulated echo. In order to obtain T2 contrast that is quite similar to SE images, the echoes must be spaced further apart, with a reduced number of echoes stimulated. However, scan time then increases.[10]

A method that uses a modified version of fast spin echo, called *DIET* (dual interval echo train), has been developed that effectively minimizes the high signal from fat without adversely affecting scan time or contrast.[11] This scheme uses an echo-train spacing at the beginning of the pulse sequence that is much longer than the ensuing echoes, to allow sufficient T2 decay of fat before subsequent data acquisition. Successive echoes are then acquired using equal and short echo-train spacing. The generated images minimize the bright signal seen from fat. Using a longer echo-train spacing for the first echo only, followed by shorter spacing, also allows for an increase in the echo-train length, which improves scan time (see Fig. 10-18).

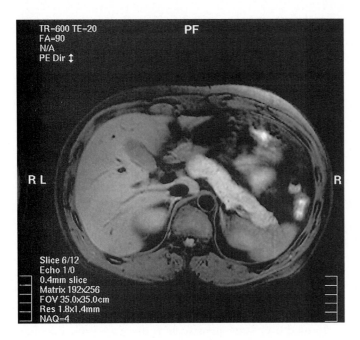

TR=600 TE=20
FA=90
N/A
PE Dir ↕

PF

R L

R

Slice 6/12
Echo 1/0
0.4mm slice
Matrix 192x256
FOV 35.0x35.0cm
Res 1.8x1.4mm
NAQ=4

Figure 10-17 Abdomen image using MSOFT. (*Courtesy Toshiba America Medical Systems, Inc. By permission.*)

A subsequent report describes a variant of the DIET technique which allows for the collection of dual echoes, the first of which is a proton-density image, often desired by the imaging team. The sequence is modified by incorporating the odd, large echo spacing in the middle of the sequence instead of at the beginning. Conventional equal and small echo-train spacing is used at the beginning of the echo train for data collection to allow for generation of a proton-density image.[12] The remaining echoes that will contribute to the T2-weighted image are acquired using a large initial echo spacing followed by smaller and equal spacing (see Fig. 10-19).

While the fat signal is not totally eliminated, it is reduced in comparison to its intensity in conventional fast spin echo images. An additional benefit of this technique is the potential for increased sensitivity to hemorrhage as a result of the increased spacing between refocusing pulses.[13]

The signal intensity of fat can have detrimental effects when obtaining MRI images for the detection of pathologic lesions. The ability to effectively minimize its signal can improve diagnostic competence. It is important

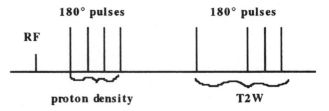

Figure 10-19 Simple graphic illustrating a variant of the DIET technique in which a proton-density image can be collected while minimizing the bright signal from fat.

to understand the techniques available for fat suppression so that they can be implemented appropriately.

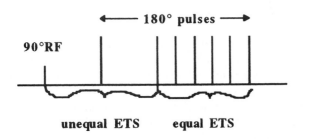

Figure 10-18 Graphic representation of the DIET scheme.

References

1. Porter BA: Overview of clinical applications of STIR.
2. Elster AD: *Questions and Answers in Magnetic Resonance Imaging.* St. Louis: Mosby, 1994.
3. Dixon WT: Simple proton spectroscopic imaging. *Radiology* 153:189–194, 1984.
4. Williams SCR, Horsfield MA, Hall LD: True water and fat MR imaging with use of multiple-echo acquisition. *Radiology* 173:249–253, 1989.
5. Young IA. Special pulse sequence and techniques, in Stark, DD, Bradley WG Jr.: *Magnetic Resonance Imaging.* St. Louis: Mosby, 1988.

6. Zhang W, Goldhaber DM, Kramer DM, Kaufman L: Separation of water and fat images at 0.35 tesla using the three-point dixon method with "sandwich" echoes. *SMR Abstract* 1995, p 656.

7. Miyazaki M, Takai H, Tokunaga Y, Hoshino T, Hanawa M: A polarity altered spectral and spatial selective acquisition technique. *SMR Abstract* 1995, p 657.

8. Miyazaki M, Kojima F, Igarashi H: Uniform fat suppression in multislice imaging: A multislice off-resonance fat suppression technique (MSOFT). *SMR Abstract* 1994, p 796.

9. Butts K, Pauly JM, Glover GH, Pelc NH: Dual echo "DIET" fast spin echo imaging. *SMR Abstract* 1995, p 651.

10. Kanazawa H, Takai H, Machida Y, Hanawa M: Contrast naturalization of fast spin echo imaging: A fat reduction technique free from field inhomogeneity. *SMR Abstract* 1994, p 494.

11. Kanazawa H, Takai H, Machida Y, Hanawa M: Contrast naturalization of fast spin echo imaging: A fat reduction technique free from field inhomogeneity. *SMR Abstract* 1994, p 494.

12. Butts K, Pauly JM, Glover GH, Pelc NH: Dual echo "DIET" fast spin echo imaging. *SMR Abstract* 1995, p 651.

13. Butts K, Pauly JM, Glover GH, Pelc NH: Dual echo "DIET" fast spin echo imaging. *SMR Abstract* 1995, p 651.

11

Functional Imaging

Functional imaging refers to methods of imaging that provide more than the anatomic or pathologic changes that are found during routine static image analysis. By definition, functional imaging implies that the activity of an organ or organ system, in addition to its appearance, is being evaluated. Examples of functional imaging that have been commonly used for some time include such techniques as nuclear medicine and ultrasound studies of the heart. Although cardiac imaging in MR has been utilized to evaluate a variety of conditions (see Chap. 19), use of MR for functional imaging of the heart and other organ systems is not yet routine. However, recent developments in rapid scan techniques (see Chap. 7) have made functional imaging more feasible.

Applications of functional imaging are being explored using the more rapid scan techniques, with which anatomic changes that occur during motion can be studied relatively easily. Kinematic studies evaluating joint motion that are processed for rapid image presentation give the final playback the appearance of actual joint function during flexion and extension. Like most cardiac applications, these images are basically a series of static images pieced together in sequence to give the added characteristic of motion. In most cases, this is a valid representation of function and provides useful information to the treating physician. Another dimension of functional imaging with MR depends on actual physiologic changes that occur during organ activity. This technique, referred to as functional magnetic resonance imaging, or FMRI, has been primarily applied to the evaluation of brain function.

Functional magnetic resonance imaging of the brain involves the detection of changes in blood volume, flow, and oxygen saturation that accompany focal activation of brain cells. That is to say, when one uses one's brain for specific functions, there are associated changes in brain metabolism that can be identified using specific MR techniques. Additional methods of evaluating such changes include positron emission tomography (PET), single photon emission computed tomography (SPECT), electroencephalography (EEG), and magnetoencephalography (MEG).

An example of the clinical utility of FMRI is in the presurgical evaluation of patients with mass lesions within the brain. When a mass, such as a brain tumor, presses on areas of the brain that control motor function, the patient will lose the ability to move some part of the body. Likewise, if an area of the brain that controls important bodily functions is removed at surgery, the patient will lose that particular function. Therefore, it is essential that the neurosurgeon not only remove the mass, but also *not* remove important functional areas of the brain. It would be beneficial, then, for the physicians caring for a patient to know not only where a brain tumor is located but, in addition, for what activity the brain next to the tumor is functionally responsible. An example is given in Figs. 11-1*A* and 11-1*B*. In this particular case, the patient has a large mass that is readily identifiable by routine MR imaging. However, the additional information provided by FMRI demonstrates the exact location of motor function (hand movement), so that the neurosurgeon not only is able to remove the brain tumor, but can also avoid removing this vital area of brain function. The methods by which such functional imaging of the brain can be accomplished using MR are somewhat varied, but they have in common techniques evaluating local changes in tissue blood flow or metabolism.

For the most part, FMRI evaluations rely upon difference images—for example, the difference between the appearance of the MR scan of a subject when the person

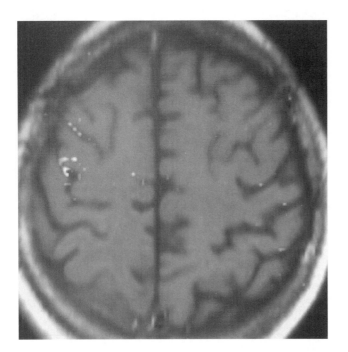

Figure 11-1A Axial GRE T1-weighted MR (TR 10, TE 4, FA 10) with FMRI data superimposed to demonstrate the location of the motor cortex *(white areas).* Compare to Fig. 11-1B.

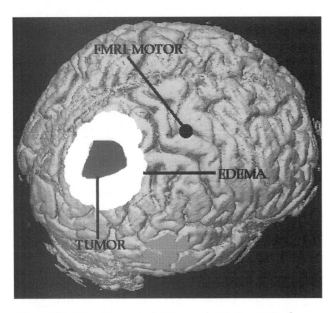

Figure 11-1B Presurgical 3D reconstruction MR demonstrating the location of this patient's brain neoplasm and surrounding edema relative to the motor cortex. This patient had significant hand weakness that resolved after surgery. Compare to Fig. 11-1A.

curred within the brain at the time that the activity was being performed (difference: Fig. 11-4). If this information is then added back onto the subject's routine scan (Fig. 11-5), the resulting "functional image" provides not only an anatomic image of the brain but the functional location of the cortical activity of the brain associated with hand movement (functional image: Fig. 11-6). In reality, it takes an average of several images with the person at rest and several images with the hand being opened and closed (in this case, 16 images of each) in order to obtain enough information to create a meaningful difference image. In other words, there is not enough change in the brain to be detected by most MR methods unless that change occurs several times and all of these trials are added together (see Figs. 11-2 to 11-4). Therefore, in this case, a total of 16 images with the person at rest were electronically "subtracted" from 16 images with the hand being opened and closed.

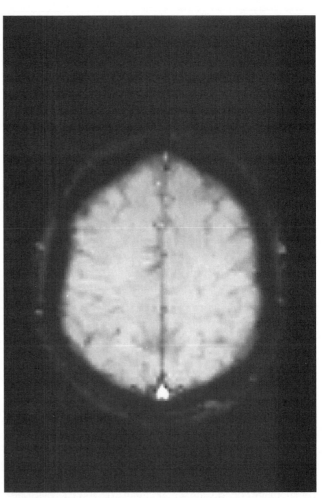

Figure 11-2 Axial GRE fast low-angle shot (FLASH) MR (TR 430, TE 50, FA 70) acquired as the "at rest" component of an FMRI study. Six slices were acquired at 5-mm thickness with a 2-mm in-plane resolution using two averages and a 128 × 128 matrix. Acquisition time for the six slices was 110 s. Compare to Figs. 11-3 and 11-4.

is at rest and this same subject's scan when an activity is being performed. If the scan of the unstimulated brain (at rest: Fig. 11-2) is electronically subtracted from the scan in the stimulated state (opening and closing the hand: Fig. 11-3), the difference image results from changes that oc-

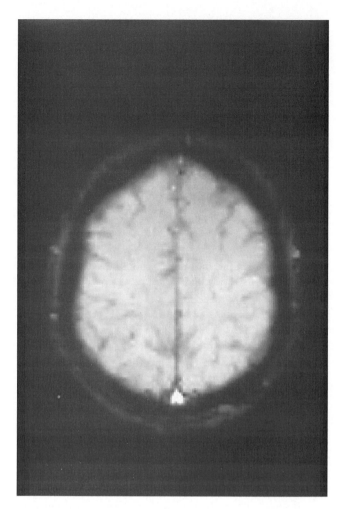

Figure 11-3 Axial GRE fast low-angle shot (FLASH) MR (TR 430, TE 50, FA 70) acquired as the "active" component of an FMRI study with the patient opening and closing the hand during the acquisition. Six slices were acquired at 5-mm thickness with a 2-mm in-plane resolution using two averages and a 128×128 matrix. Acquisition time for the six slices was 110 s. Compare to Figs. 11-2 and 11-4. Note that there is no apparent difference between this image and the one in Fig. 11-2; however, the difference image in Fig. 11-4 shows that there is a measurable change.

The exact nature of the changes in the brain that are being measured is the subject of some controversy in the MR literature. The first functional images of the brain using MR relied upon bolus injections of gadolinium. Clearly, the dominant activity measured in these studies was the changes related to local cerebral blood volume (CBV) and/or regional cerebral blood flow (CBF). Both CBV and CBF are known from PET studies to change when local areas of the brain are active. It is also known that this focal brain cell activation or neuronal activity results in changes in blood oxygenation. Gadolinium is not required to visualize changes in blood oxygenation that accompany changes in regional CBV and CBF. Therefore,

imaging sequences have been designed to exploit these types of localized changes in brain metabolism.

As the brain uses oxygen, the blood loses oxygen, and there is a buildup of deoxyhemoglobin within the venous blood. Deoxyhemoglobin has a fairly strong paramagnetic effect (similar to that of gadolinium), at least at higher field strengths (1.0 and 1.5 teslas or higher). Therefore, gadolinium is not required in order to measure changes in oxygen usage by the brain. However, all is not as it may at first seem. This is because when we use the brain, we also significantly increase the CBV and CBF to the area of the brain being used—so much so, in fact, that there is a net increase in local oxygenation. This results in a net decrease in the amount of deoxyhemoglobin, so that the difference image obtained actually represents a *loss* of deoxyhemoglobin or an *increase* in oxygen.

Although gadolinium-enhanced methods of functional MR were first used, nonenhanced techniques are now more typically preferred. Since the signal on MR is altered by changes in blood oxygenation, the term *blood-*

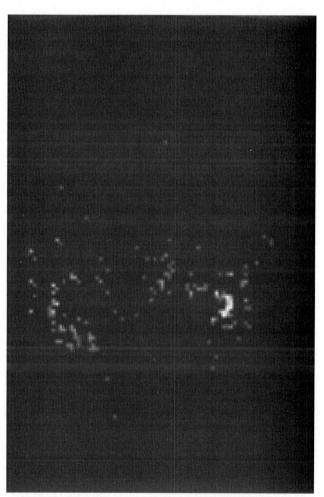

Figure 11-4 "Difference image" between Figs. 11-2 and 11-3. Note that there is an area that is significantly brighter on this computer-subtracted study, representing the region of motor cortex "activated" by opening and closing the hand.

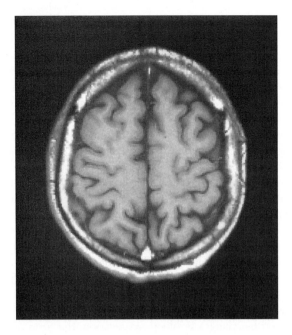

Figure 11-5   Axial GRE T1-weighted MR (TR 10, TE 4, FA 10) without FMRI data superimposed. This represents the "template" upon which the functional data will be superimposed. Compare to Fig. 11-6.

oxygen-level-dependent, or BOLD, was coined to describe this type of naturally occurring contrast effect. Therefore, in functional MR, BOLD techniques are usually employed as the method of contrast that takes advantage of natural tissue differences which occur when the brain is functioning. This form of imaging does not measure neu-

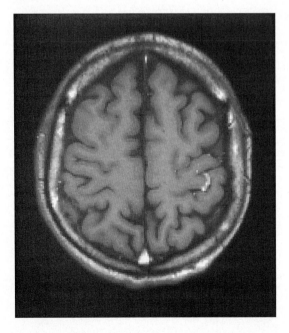

Figure 11-6   Axial GRE T1-weighted MR (TR 10, TE 4, FA 10) with FMRI data superimposed to demonstrate the location of the motor cortex *(white areas).* This represents a computer superimposition of Figs. 11-4 and 11-5.

ronal activity directly, but rather is an indirect measure of the brain's activation. Even though it is not currently possible to directly relate the MR signal changes that are observed to the amount of brain cell activity, by using two acquisitions obtained under different neurologically active conditions, relative oxygenation differences can be mapped on MR images to create FMRI techniques.

FMRI, then, is based on seeing MR signal differences between two acquisitions obtained at points in time of differing neuronal activity. The most common form of difference in neuronal activity is between some type of stimulation and the normal resting state—for example, a simple lights on and lights off type of stimulation. The FMRI would measure the difference in the brain's response to the conditions of rest and body movement. It would be anticipated that there would be activation of the cortex when the movement occurs and minimal activity in this part of the brain is at rest.

The technical demands of FMRI are among the greatest encountered in MR imaging; however, the studies can be viewed in terms of imaging sequences that are in general well known. These are the familiar methods of spin echo (SE) and gradient recalled echo (GRE). In addition, a further distinction can be made between slow and fast imaging techniques. The "slow" methods include fast low-angle shot (FLASH) GRE and standard SE, while the fast techniques are represented by echo planar imaging (EPI).

The choice of imaging sequences depends in part on equipment availability, and in addition upon the information desired. There is a significant body of evidence to suggest that SE signals arise from tissue capillaries, but that GRE signals come from both capillaries and larger veins. FMRI methods in general place tremendous temporal demands on MR equipment.

EPI may be necessary in order to effectively speed up FMRI SE acquisitions. EPI methods use specialized gradient and data acquisition hardware to allow for a full image in about 1 s using an echo time of 14 to 60 ms. Even though the actual image can be acquired in as little as 20 to 100 ms, a delay between image acquisitions is necessary for the recovery of longitudinal magnetization, and this increases the effective imaging time to approximately 1 s.

GRE FLASH sequences are usually available, at least in a single-slice technique, that allow for image acquisition in the range of 3 to 10 s. Although the neuronal response that is being localized occurs on a scale of 10 to 100 ms, the accompanying physiologic changes in blood flow and metabolism that are being measured by techniques such as FMRI, PET, and SPECT occur over several seconds. Therefore, these slower imaging times are effective for the slower metabolic changes that are actually being evaluated. That is, the brain cells work very, very fast, but the changes in blood and tissue chemistry that accompany this brain cell activity are relatively slow.

Therefore, no matter how fast you image in MR, you are still measuring a somewhat slow event. There is no current MR technique that can look directly at brain cell activity, even though there are MR scan techniques that can image at the same speed as neuronal activity. Nonetheless, evaluating these secondary responses is important in advancing our understanding of the brain in both the normal and abnormal states.

Signal-to-noise ratio (SNR) issues arise in FMRI just as they do in all other areas of MR imaging. EPI is effective in terms of SNR as well as temporal considerations, since a 40-ms EPI image will be comparable in SNR to a 2-s FLASH image. In addition to EPI, current FMRI techniques also benefit from increasing magnetic field strength and active shielded gradient coils that will reduce eddy currents. Coil choices are similar to those for other types of MR imaging, in that typically the improved SNR provided by a specialized surface coil with limited field of view (FOV) must be balanced against the desire for the larger FOV that is available when using a whole head coil.

The sequence parameters that are chosen in FMRI include TR, TE, and flip angle, just as in routine MR imaging. However, unlike in standard clinical imaging, the goal is not to maximize general tissue contrast, but to improve contrast with respect to changes in susceptibility and deoxyhemoglobin levels.

Experimental evidence suggests that the ideal TE for FMRI is in the range of 30 to 40 ms, and that a TR of approximately 70 with a flip angle of 40° can be effectively used for visualization experiments such as the one described above. The flip angle (FA) used in FLASH GRE examinations is chosen in order to maximize signal strength while limiting inflow sensitivity from blood (see Figs. 11-3 and 11-4). This provides an effective compromise between SNR and susceptibility weighting, since both SE and GRE susceptibility-induced signal alterations increase with increasing TE. Not only is the choice of TE

important from the standpoint of susceptibility changes, but it also determines the amount of time required to obtain a phase-encoded line. TE, then, determines the number of spatial slices, the image phase-encoded lines, the TR, and imaging speed.

The number of slices required for an FMRI study depends on the necessary amount of anatomic coverage and the desired temporal resolution. The anatomic coverage needed is often dependent upon the amount of uncertainty regarding the location of the brain activity being evaluated. Ideally, the entire brain would be studied, with the location of activity being determined by the resulting images. For the most part, however, this is currently a practical impossibility. Therefore, in most instances, it is necessary to pick a region of interest to be evaluated by FMRI. The availability of EPI, however, allows for entire head coverage using 3D imaging in approximately 2 s. This allows for the study of bilateral activations as well as the identification of supplementary regions of brain activity.

There are, in effect, a diverse number of sequence requirements for FMRI. These include consideration of susceptibility weighting, image stability, imaging speed, and sensitivity to artifacts. EPI appears to effectively address each of these issues, and as the hardware for EPI is becoming more commonly available, FMRI will no doubt be more frequently utilized.

Suggested Reading

Orrison WW Jr, Lewine JD, Sander JA, Hartshorne MF: *Functional Brain Imaging.* St. Louis, MO, Mosby, 1995.

12

Artifact-Suppression Techniques

Each day the changes in our physical orientation, and the direction and speed of our movement through life, are not unlike what is occurring inside of our bodies. Our bodies have a variety of moving fluids flowing through well-defined tubes: cerebral spinal fluid, lymphatic fluid, un-oxygenated blood within veins, oxygenated blood in arteries, capillary blood, and bile, all having a constant velocity, albeit different from one another. In addition to fluid movement, physiologic conditions such as respiration, peristalsis, and cardiac motion are necessary for viability. These moving spins wreak havoc on our MR images, causing artifacts that may obliterate an area of interest. It has long been realized that in order to obtain the most accurate information on structures within the body, we need to compensate for the motion generated by these activities.

The intent of this chapter is to identify the compensatory means available to the MR operator to reduce artifacts caused by physiologic motion, thus maximizing image quality. Many techniques exist today that, when used properly, can greatly influence the quality of MR images. This chapter will discuss in detail the methods currently available, the mechanisms behind their function, and the importance of their use in imaging sequences. In addition, a discussion on the effect that gradient magnetic fields have on spin phases will be included.

The Effect of Gradients on Spin Phase Changes

The phase of a process relates a point in its cycle to a point in time. If two processes are at the same point in the cycle, they will be doing the same thing. The effect of motion on the MR images is a result of the spin phase differences that result from the movement of the spins while under the influence of a gradient magnetic field. During the course of an acquisition, imaging gradients are applied repeatedly in all spatial dimensions. When they are applied, an accumulation of phase shift (net gain or loss of phase angle) is induced in spins that are moving. Any coordinate (X, Y, or Z dimension) that has a velocity component that is not zero, such as the moving spins of blood flow in the superior/inferior (Z-coordinate) direction, can have a phase shift induced in the spin. Stationary tissues have a velocity component that is zero; therefore, no phase shift is identified (see Fig. 12-1). For the phase-encoding coordinate, this is expected and necessary. However, for slice and frequency-encoding coordinates, this poses a problem.

It has long been recognized that phase shift depends upon the position, velocity, and acceleration of a spin as well as upon the strength and polarity with which a gradient magnetic field is applied. The progression of momentum or force ("order of moment") of the gradient magnetic field with respect to time is described in terms of contribution to phase shift, where position is related to zeroth order, velocity is related to first order, and acceleration is related to second order.

Three well-known effects of spin phase shifts on the appearance of the MR image are documented:

1. *Intravoxel phase dispersion, resulting in darkening of the signal.* Flow velocity has a parabolic profile (laminar) across the lumen of the vessel. The velocity in the center of the lumen is fast, whereas that closer to the periphery is slow. The overall effect is a velocity that is not constant. The distribution of these spin velocities within a voxel produces a phase dispersion when veloc-

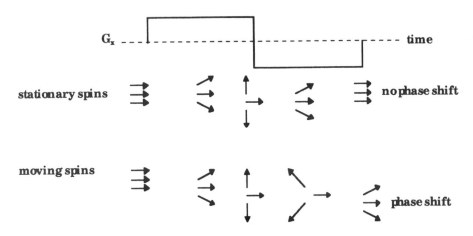

Figure 12-1   Spins in the presence of a bipolar gradient magnetic field.

ity changes by about 1 cm/s or more. The resulting intravoxel signal is greatly reduced.

2. *Even-echo rephasing of the first-order motion.* It has been observed that the signal from some blood vessels appears brighter on second echoes, even though T2 decay predicts a decrease in signal intensity with time. This phenomenon is related to the use of bipolar refocusing pulses in which the amplitude of the gradient is equal in the positive and negative directions, as seen in Fig. 12-1. These bipolar gradients will refocus only the spins of stationary tissues. The spins that are moving will have a net phase loss. The signal for the first, odd echo is dark. Subsequently, this loss can be unintentionally reversed on even echoes if the refocusing pulse is paired to the 180° RF pulse. This results from the addition of symmetric gradient pulses with lobe polarities that are reversed from the normal positive gradient. The second, even-echo signal intensity appears bright (see Fig. 12-2). This phenomenon holds true for odd/even echo sequences in which linear gradients are applied symmetrically around the 180° RF pulse. Only first-order motion (velocity) is rephased.

3. *Misregistration of flow signal as a result of pulsation of blood and CSF.* The pulsatile nature of CSF and arterial flow sometimes produces ghost images across the imaging plane along the phase-encoding direction (see Fig. 12-3). This occurs because data collection is implemented during the timed procedure of the pulse sequence (TR-dependent) and cardiac cycle of individuals. The cardiac cycle can vary tremendously from patient to patient, producing blood velocity that is inconsistent in terms of phase-shift expectations.

The consequence of these phenomena is seen in the final product. The results emanate from spins or groups of protons that move at different velocities within a magnetic field. They will experience changes in precessional frequency and phase at different rates. Consequently, they will dephase more rapidly. This is in addition to the normal loss of phase coherence as a result of T2 effects. When the pulse sequence is not designed to adequately rephase the moving spins, moving blood will be mapped in the wrong location in the phase direction. The artifact can be traced to its origination (i.e., the blood vessel it is coming from). It is inconsistent in signal intensity, appearing bright at one location yet black at another, depending on its direction and velocity. This artifact may be misinterpreted as a lesion or may cause generalized image degradation. In the best interests of a correct diagnosis, it needs to be compensated; it is irrelevant whether there is a

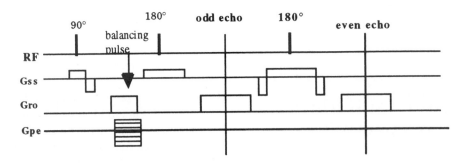

Figure 12-2   Spin echo pulse sequence diagram showing balancing and refocusing pulses. G_{ss} = slice select gradient; G_{ro} = readout gradient; G_{pe} = phase-encoding gradient.

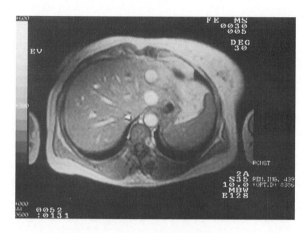

Figure 12-3   Axial abdomen shows typical ghosting pattern seen as a result of the pulsatile nature of the aorta.

bright signal within the vessel or whether there is a signal void. However, we want the signal to be accurately located in the final image. We accomplish this task by using unique pulse sequences that are sensitive to phase changes of moving spins. In some instances, a simple change in the way the pulse sequence is acquired accomplishes the same task, with few trade-offs.

The artifact-suppression techniques discussed in this chapter are commonly used to minimize or eliminate motion artifacts caused by physiologic processes that are not under operator control.

Reorientation of Phase- and Frequency-Encoding Directions

During data acquisition, information is collected in three coordinates to spatially define the object dimensionally. Using all three gradient coil pairs, projections of a two-dimensional image are created from a three-dimensional object.

Patient movement and flow in arteries, veins, and the subarachnoid space cause artifactual representations on the MR image. When the data are collected, they contain information with regard to the phase, frequency, and amplitude of the signal. This is based on the original position of the spins in the phase direction. The spins, however, move, and will not be at the original location at the end of the acquisition. Since phase information is collected a multitude of times at distinct intervals, there is a phase shift that will cause the spins' signal to be mismapped in the phase-encoding direction. Essentially, the spins that

had originally absorbed RF energy at the beginning of the pulse sequence are no longer available to reemit the energy, and a flow artifact is generated. The artifact will be seen as a result of the gradients' failure to completely eliminate the phase contribution of either the slice select or frequency-encoding gradient when motion occurs in these planes.

Phase-versus-frequency reorientation is a simple procedure with no time or image quality penalties, if used in its pure state. It is an operator-selectable maneuver which offers artifact control by merely swapping the orientation of phase versus frequency. By directing phase encoding in a different direction, flow and motion artifacts can be minimized. They are never completely eliminated, but are reduced to a more tolerable level.

An example of phase-versus-frequency orientation can help to illustrate this. Consider the situation of imaging the lumbar spine using a sagittal projection, with phase encoding directed anterior to posterior. Vascular flow is predominantly in the superior-to-inferior direction, while respiratory motion in general is anterior-to-posterior, and peristalsis is random. Cardiac motion occurs in various orientations as well. A generalized streaking artifact can be seen, propagating anterior to posterior on an uncompensated image (see Fig. 12-4). This occurs because every time the abdomen or thorax moves, the tissue spins will be in a different location. For each phase-encoding step, a phase shift will occur, so that at the end of the acquisition a cumulative effect of shifts will be rendered to create the final image.

When the phase-encoding direction is changed to run superior to inferior, in this example, the chance of minimizing phase shift is greater because the spins in blood are running generally in the same direction. Additionally, less motion occurs to produce the artifact (see Fig. 12-5).

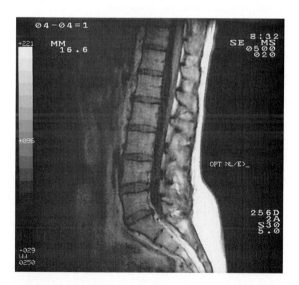

Figure 12-4   Sagittal lumbar spine reveals generalized streaking in the A-P direction.

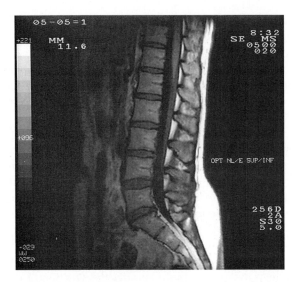

Figure 12-5   Sagittal lumbar spine on same patient as in Fig. 12-4 shows significantly reduced streaking artifact when phase direction is S-I.

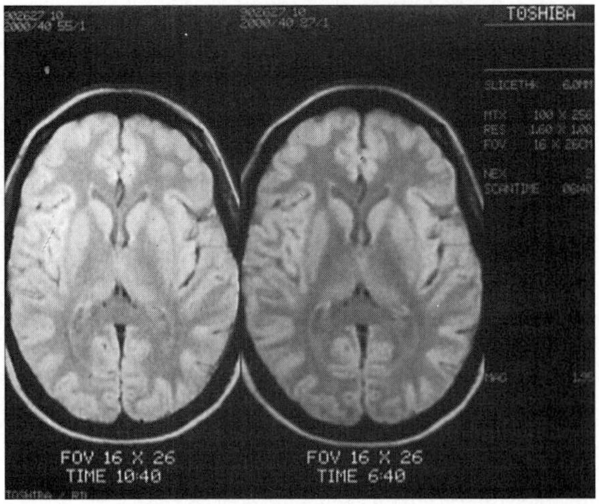

Figure 12-6   The transaxial brain image on the right was acquired with PE direction L-R and a reduced matrix. The image on the left used a 256 × 256 matrix with an A-P direction.

When selecting the phase-versus-frequency orientation for the imaging procedure, care must be used to ensure that aliasing artifact is not inadvertently produced. In our example above, if the phase-encoding direction is changed from A-P without a commensurate change in FOV to accommodate the added dimension, aliasing can result.

In some cases, reorienting phase and frequency allows the operator to tailor the number of phase-encoding steps to an anatomic region that is small, thus reducing scan time (see Fig. 12-6). Spatial resolution is decreased as a direct result of reducing the number of phase-encoding steps per fixed FOV, resulting in fewer pixels per matrix that are larger (see Chaps. 4 and 5). Signal-to-noise ratio per pixel will increase, however.

Table 12-1 identifies the common slice select, phase-encoding, and frequency-encoding directions for conventional MR imagers. Refer to the operator's manual for the system you are using for further guidance.

Phase-encoding direction can be identified using observed motion artifacts as a guide. Since motion is always visible in the phase-encoding direction, the operator need only identify the direction of motion to distinguish the gradient pair used for encoding that orientation.

Antialiasing Techniques

When an anatomical region of interest exceeds the field of view chosen by the operator, an artifact called *aliasing* or *wraparound* occurs. Aliasing may also occur as a result of pulsatile flow (e.g., in the popliteal artery), which is seen as signal exceeding the FOV. The artifact is a result of signal being mismapped on the final image on the opposite side of the matrix. See Chap. 6 for a complete discussion of aliasing artifacts.

Antialiasing techniques are available in most system software in the readout or frequency direction and the

TABLE 12-1 ENCODING GRADIENT IDENTIFICATION ON CONVENTIONAL IMAGERS

Spatial Encoding	Transaxial (S-I)	Sagittal (L-R)	Coronal (A-P)
Slice selection	Z gradient	X gradient	Y gradient
Phase encoding	Y gradient	Y gradient	X gradient
Frequency encoding	X gradient	Z gradient	Z gradient

S-I: superior to inferior—Z direction of magnet
A-P: anterior to posterior—Y direction of magnet
L-R: left to right—X direction of magnet

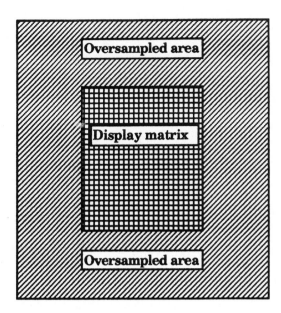

Figure 12-7 Antiphase/antifrequency technique in which both acquisition matrices are doubled. The oversampled area is ignored during reconstruction, so that the final image is that of the actual matrix selections.

phase-encoding direction. This technique involves oversampling the data during acquisition, then ignoring signal from the oversampled area, which is outside the region of interest (see Fig. 12-7). The final image is reconstructed using data collected from the selected display matrix.

The use of antialiasing techniques does not affect display resolution. That is, if a 256×256 matrix is chosen using antialiasing techniques (data are collected using a 512×512 acquisition matrix), the final image is reconstructed with only 256 rows of phase containing 256 data samples. Thus, the resolution is that of a 1-mm by 1-mm pixel.

Oversampling in the readout direction does not affect imaging time, since the frequency-encoding function is not a factor in the scan-time equation. It will, however, affect the number of slices available per TR, since the time necessary to collect extra data points increases the minimum TR per slice.

Oversampling in the phase-encoding direction does induce a time penalty by a factor of 2. This may be compensated for by decreasing the number of acquisitions proportionally without a loss in signal.

Double matrix methods of oversampling result in images without aliased artifacts (see Fig. 12-8). This has the overall effect of improving signal-to-noise ratio by decreasing the noise component associated with the artifact. When performed with half the number of acquisitions normally used for the sequence, there is no time penalty and the signal-to-noise ratio is not compromised.

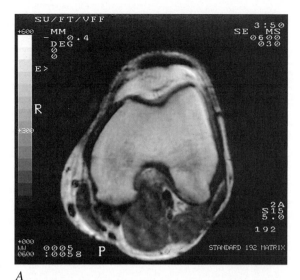

A

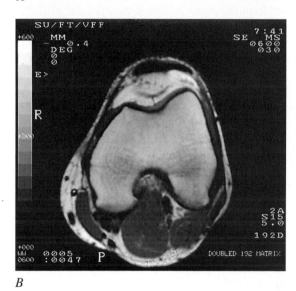

B

Figure 12-8 Axial knee shows loss of detail caused by subtle wraparound artifact resulting from popliteal flow artifact (posteriorly) and coupling from contact with the coil by the opposite knee. There is a dramatic decrease in the artifact when antialiasing technique in the form of a double PE matrix is used. Since the number of acquisitions was kept constant, scan time doubled.

Presaturation Techniques

Presaturation is used to eliminate signal that results from moving spins, preventing it from entering the scan region and producing an artifact. To accomplish this, additional RF pulses are applied to regions adjacent to the image volume of interest. Using conventional presaturation techniques, the RF pulse in megahertz is usually that of the

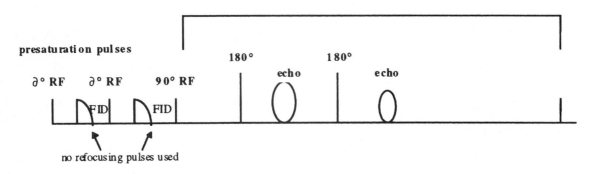

Conventional Spin Echo Pulse Sequence

presaturation pulses

∂° RF   ∂° RF   90° RF   180°   echo   180°   echo

FID   FID

no refocusing pulses used

Figure 12-9 SE pulse sequence using two presaturation bands. The FID signal is not refocused, so that the spins will not produce a signal.

center frequency and is written as a portion of the pulse sequence being performed (see Fig. 12-9).

In sequences using magnetization transfer methods of saturation, a specific frequency is applied that will selectively excite the hydrogen associated with macromolecules, such as protein, thus lowering the relaxation time of free water (see Fig. 12-10). The net result is an improvement in tissue contrast, such as that of blood vessels, by increased saturation of parenchyma. This concept is described in detail in Chap. 9.

When moving spins from blood are exposed to quick, repetitive RF pulses, they are never allowed to recover any longitudinal magnetization; therefore, they are never able to generate a signal. When the image acquisition is performed, moving spins that have been presaturated do not contribute to the overall SNR. Only those spins within the imaging volume generate a signal. Consequently, artifact from blood flow is minimized.

Presaturation can be accomplished in the direction of the slice or perpendicular to the slice. When presaturation is to be performed perpendicular to the slice plane, operator-selectable bands are placed according to the region

to be saturated. This is sometimes referred to as in-plane presaturation.

In-plane presaturation is a technique that reduces signal adjacent to the scanned area of interest. The use of in-plane presaturation in a sagittal lumbar spine image will reduce artifacts caused by flow and peristalsis that would affect the spinal column and spinal canal. In sagittal cervical spine imaging, the signal from the motion of the epiglottis, tongue, and mandible can be reduced.

Presaturation bands that are applied in the direction of the slice are useful in transaxial imaging, since most blood flow occurs vertically (head to foot) in the patient. The potential for artifactual signal produced by moving spins is eliminated because free induction decay is not reversed, and therefore no signal is produced (see Fig. 12-11).

The flip angle used for the presaturation RF pulses is operator-selectable in most cases. It can be chosen to optimize saturation by the spins. Increasing the flip angle has a saturation effect on spins, so that flip angles between 90° and 120° generally are used to provide adequate saturation.

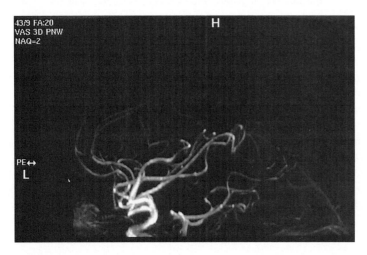

43/9 FA:20
VAS 3D PNW
NAQ=2

H

PE↔
L

Figure 12-10 MR vascular image using magnetization transfer technique in the form of slice-selective off-resonance sinc pulse (SORS) to increase visualization of peripheral vessels. This is in addition to conventional presaturation to minimize signal from veins. (*Courtesy Toshiba America Medical Systems, Inc. By permission.*)

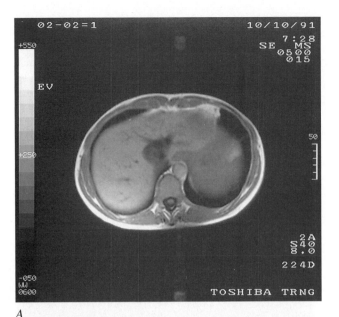

A

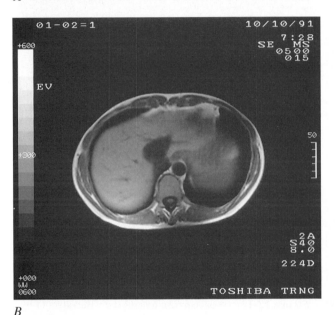

B

Figure 12-11 *(A)* Axial abdomen image at level of upper abdomen shows ghosting artifact from aortic flow. *(B)* This image was produced using two presaturation bands, one placed superior to the FOV, the other inferior. Flow artifacts are not visible.

In many MR imagers, the selection of presaturation bands allows manipulation of the size of the band as well as the number of bands permissible by the system. The size of the band has an effect on the amount of spins whose signals are reduced (see Fig. 12-12). The larger the band, the less signal will be represented in the area of the presaturation band because more spins are saturated.

Band placement is critical for several reasons. If the RF pulse applied is not "clean," a form of contamination occurs in which the edge of the presaturation band is uneven and appears to "bleed" into areas of desired signal.

This has been termed *roll-off* by some investigators. It can affect image quality by reducing signal in areas where maximum signal and contrast are necessary. It is occasionally necessary to place the band further from the artifact-producing area than would normally be the case. For example, when anterior presaturation band placement in the abdomen is used to minimize signal from the aorta for imaging of the lumbar spine, the presaturation band should be positioned to cover as much of the artery as possible, since the aorta is located fairly close to the vertebral body. If roll-off exists, saturation can inadvertently occur in the vertebral body as well.

An important argument against the use of presaturation bands is that the lack of signal from anatomic regions may prevent evaluation of an area that could in fact contain pathology. Each site should consider the benefits of presaturation bands versus the disadvantages of eliminating signals from large areas of anatomy.

The use of saturation bands will increase RF power deposition to the patient by the application of additional RF pulses. Energy in the form of watts of power is increased with an increase in flip angle as well. So when multiple presaturation bands are used with relatively high flip angles, SAR (specific absorption rate) levels to the patient are increased. Furthermore, the use of presaturation bands with most fast scan techniques, such as fast spin echo and fast IR, will significantly increase RF power deposition, and so a reduction in slices per TR is inevitable. Most MR manufacturers limit the number of slices per TR when using presaturation bands by automatically reducing the number of slices. In some cases, coverage must be obtained by increasing the number of data sets collected, increasing the slice thickness and/or gap, or increasing the TR.

Table 12-2 describes the effect on flow artifacts, respiratory motion, and peristalsis that placement of presaturation bands affords. Remember that at the aortic arch, flow from arteries moves superior toward the head and inferior toward the feet. Presaturation-band placement and its effect will be dependent on the level of the imaging plane relative to the direction of flow of the vessel.

Flow Compensation — Gradient Moment Nulling Technique

Flow compensation is a method that uses a gradient moment nulling technique to eliminate or reduce artifacts caused by phase accumulation of moving spins.

When spins move while a gradient is on, they accu-

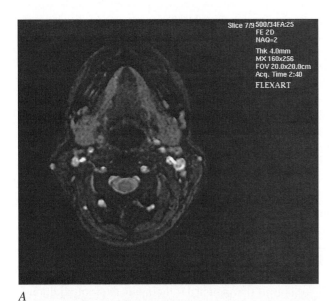

A

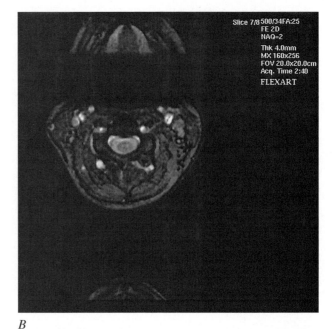

B

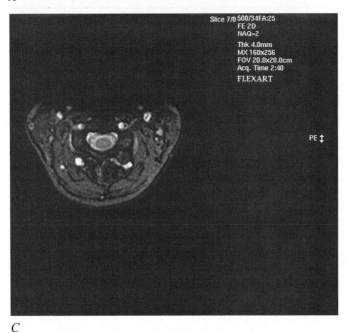

C

Figure 12-12   Axial cervical images show the effect of presaturation-band size on image quality. Note the increase in T2 contrast in CSF on image *(C)* with the use of a wide presaturation band.

mulate a phase shift. This is why you see the flow artifact in the phase-encoding direction. In sagittal imaging of the knee, for example, blood flow in the popliteal artery causes artifacts that can reduce the visibility of the anatomy in the joint. Blood flow can also mask pathology in the posterior aspect of the leg.

In order to understand the mechanism behind gradient moment nulling techniques, it is important to understand the condition of a moment. In the discussion of phase changes found earlier in this chapter, the moment was described as the force or momentum of the spins produced by the gradient magnetic fields. There are many "orders" of moments. The first is related to the position of the object

(spin); we call this "zeroth order." The progression of moments advances with increasing complexity. If there is a change in position, velocity has occurred; this is called "first-order moment." A change in velocity is known as acceleration and is termed "second-order moment." As the spin movement becomes more complex, such as during turbulence or pulsatility, higher orders of moments exist.

In the equations below, an attempt is made to clarify the relationship between spin phases and gradient applications. The position of a moving spin at time t can be expressed using Eq. (12.1):

$$x(t) = x_0 + vt + \tfrac{1}{2}at^2 \qquad (12.1)$$

TABLE 12-2 PRESATURATION BAND EFFECT ON PHYSIOLOGIC MOTION

Areas	Locator	Plane	Band Position	Effect
Brain	Sagittal	Axial, coronal	Superior	Venous flow
			Inferior	Arterial flow
	Coronal	Sagittal	Superior	Venous flow
			Inferior	Arterial flow
Pituitary	Coronal	Sagittal	Inferior	Arterial flow
			Superior	Venous flow
			Posterior	Venous flow, CSF
	Sagittal	Coronal	Inferior	Arterial flow
			Superior	Venous flow
			Posterior	Venous flow, CSF
Cervical spine	Sagittal	Axial, coronal	Superior	Venous flow
			Inferior	Arterial flow
	Sagittal	Sagittal, axial	Anterior	Swallowing, movement of mandible, tongue
Thoracic spine	Sagittal	Axial, coronal	Inferior	Venous flow
			Superior	Arterial and venous flow
	Sagittal	Sagittal	Anterior	Cardiac and respiratory motion
			Superior	Arterial and venous flow
			Inferior	Venous flow
Lumbar spine	Sagittal	Axial, coronal, sagittal	Anterior	Peristalsis and respirations
			Superior	Arterial flow
			Inferior	Venous flow
Liver	Sagittal	Axial, coronal, sagittal	Anterior	Respiratory motion
			Superior	Arterial flow
			Inferior	Venous flow
Knee	Coronal	Axial, sagittal	Superior	Arterial flow
			Inferior	Venous flow
	Sagittal	Coronal	Superior	Arterial flow
			Inferior	Venous flow
Shoulder	Axial	Coronal, sagittal	Medial	Respirations, arterial flow
			Inferior	Antialiasing from arm
Elbow	Coronal	Axial, sagittal	Superior	Arterial flow
	Sagittal	Coronal	Superior	Arterial flow

Here x_0 is the original position of the moving spin, v is its velocity, and a is its acceleration. The phase shift $\Delta\phi$ that the spin accumulates while under the influence of a gradient $G_x(t)$ is proportional:

$$\Delta\phi \propto \int_0^T G_x(t)x(t)\, dt \qquad (12.2)$$

If we substitute Eq. (12.1) for $x(t)$ into the expression for phase shift, we come up with the following:

$$\Delta\phi \propto \int_0^T G_x(t)\left(x_0 + vt + \tfrac{1}{2}at^2\right) dt \qquad (13.3)$$

Separating out the terms of the equation, we find

$$\Delta\phi \propto \int_0^T G_x(t)x_0\, dt + \int_0^T G_x(t)vt\, dt + \tfrac{1}{2}\int_0^T G_x(t)at^2\, dt \qquad (13.4)$$

Note that the first term is dependent on the position x_0, the second term is dependent on the velocity v, and the

third term is dependent on the acceleration a. This last equation shows that the phase shift depends upon the position, velocity, and acceleration of the spin. Each term of the equation represents a different moment of the gradient field. The goal of designing the sequence is to use the gradients to minimize the contribution of each term, since the gradient is the only thing we can control. If phase shift can be reduced to zero by choosing the appropriate gradient, then that gradient moment will have been nulled or reduced.

This is accomplished through the use of additional gradients that are applied during the pulse sequence, in essence to force the moving spins to a phase location that existed prior to acquisition. Gradient waveforms can be designed to control temporal moments by highlighting the contribution of specified spin characteristics and eliminating others. By carefully tailoring gradient pulse design, zeroth-, first-, and second-order moments can be reduced significantly. All gradient moments with the exception of phase encoding should be compensated. This requires

Figure 12-13 Simple pulse sequence diagram identifies phase dispersion as it relates to gradient application. The objective is to have no phase dispersion at the time of data collection. *Gss* = slice select gradient; *Gro* = readout gradient; *Gpe* = phase-encoding gradient; φ o = phase dispersion.

more sophisticated gradient waveforms, which are often associated with delay in echo time, and therefore additional T2 decay. Figure 12-13 represents a typical gradient waveform used in the slice select direction. In practice, additional gradient reversals are added about the RO gradients to compensate for motion artifact when it occurs in that direction.

Gradient moment nulling is a technique that increases immunity to motion in general. It helps to compensate for *any* physiologic movement. Flow-compensated sequences are especially useful in anatomic regions where CSF and blood flow are prominent, such as the posterior fossa, knee, or spine. The appearance of the image is improved as a result of an indirect increase in SNR and contrast resulting from a reduction in noise (artifact). Blood vessels will be bright, and they will be in the proper position in the final image (see Fig. 12-14).

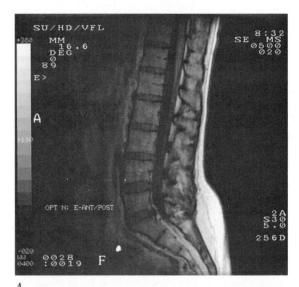

A

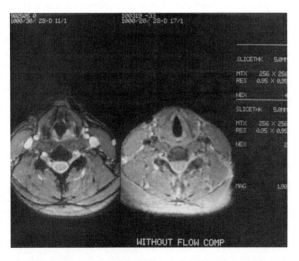

Figure 12-14 Axial cervical spine images representing flow-compensated and non-flow-compensated techniques. The image on the right shows flow artifact A-P and general image quality degradation. The image on the left used flow compensation in the slice and readout directions. Blood vessels appear bright.

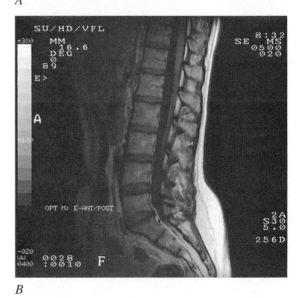

B

Figure 12-15 *A.* Sagittal lumbar spine image using conventional SE technology with no flow compensation. *B.* narrow-bandwidth sequence has flow compensation in the readout direction. Phase direction on both scans was A-P.

There are disadvantages associated with this pulse sequence. Because of the complicated waveforms of flow-compensated sequences, a longer TE is required, which means there is a greater T2 decay. In addition, because of the longer TEs used, the number of slices per TR may be reduced. The reason for this lies in the fact that during any one pulse sequence, several functions are being performed which require the use of gradient coils. These include slice selection, phase encoding, and frequency encoding or readout. When flow compensation is applied, more gradient functions are added. The TR is the same as before, however, more functions are performed during that TR time. This limits the number of slices the system can gather.

Flow-compensation techniques do not directly affect scan time. Scan time is a function of TR time, the number of phase-encoding steps, and the number of times the data are collected (acquisitions). In some cases, such as in 3DFT imaging, the number of slices also affects scan time. However, since the number of slices per TR is usually diminished using flow-compensation methods, the operator may be required to increase the TR in order to add slices to obtain the necessary coverage. Only then would scan time be increased relative to using a flow-compensation technique.

Flow compensation can be used with other artifact-suppression techniques. However, remember that whenever additional gradient applications or RF pulses are

TABLE 12-3 FLOW-COMPENSATION TIPS

Part	Vessels	Needs	Slice	Phase	Readout
Brain	Internal carotid artery, dural sinuses	• Compensation needed in both slice and readout directions. • Use presaturation in the neck to further eliminate flow artifacts.	Axial	Anterior-posterior	Left-right
Brain	Internal carotid arteries, vertebral arteries, dural sinuses	• Readout compensation most important; needs second-order compensation. • Use presaturation in the neck to further eliminate flow artifacts.	Coronal	Left-right	Inferior-superior
Brain	Dural sinuses will cause most artifacts	• Slice compensation most important. • Use of short TE (T1-weighted exams) will aid artifact reduction.	Sagittal	Inferior-superior	Anterior-posterior
Lumbar spine and cervical spine	Abdominal aorta, inferior vena cava, miscellaneous abdominal vessels	• Readout direction most important direction; must match direction of flow. • Slice compensation not required for sagittal spine. • Saturation of anterior abdomen necessary to reduce artifacts from breathing and peristalsis.	Sagittal	Anterior-posterior	Inferior-superior
Lumbar spine and cervical spine	Abdominal aorta, inferior vena cava, miscellaneous abdominal vessels	• Slice compensation most important. • Phase A-P if peristalsis not a problem. • Reduce all abdominal artifacts with saturation anterior and lateral.	Axial	Anterior-posterior	Left-right
Knee	Popliteal artery	• Readout direction most important. • Saturation above knee to further reduce flow artifacts.	Sagittal	Anterior-posterior	Inferior-superior
Knee	Popliteal artery	• Readout direction most important. • Saturation above knee to further reduce flow artifacts.	Coronal	Left-right	Inferior-superior

added to a sequence, the number of slices per TR diminishes. Also, RF power deposition to the patient may increase, further limiting the number of slices.

Any gradient can be used to create a well-behaved gradient moment. In general, the gradient moment reduction is performed using the slice select and readout gradient. The process of phase encoding calls for a phase shift in that direction, so we don't necessarily want to compensate. The trick for the operator is to choose the flow-compensated pulse sequence that will have the greatest benefit in the imaging plane of interest (see Fig. 12-15). That means that the technologist must be able to identify the anatomy and direction of flow of the vasculature within the imaging volume. The flow-compensation sequence must then be chosen to minimize the effects of those phase-shifted spins. Table 12-3 can be used as a reference guide to help identify the most appropriate use of flow-compensated sequences for an imaging system. It is not intended to cover all body parts, imaging needs, or system features. It is, however, intended to make you aware that decisions regarding phase-encoding direction should take flow-compensation needs into account. Familiarity with the sequence designs of the imaging system you are using will ultimately help in selecting the proper flow-compensated sequence for the imaging purpose.

The table takes into account the direction of the most artifact-producing flow, slice plane, and body part. When planning a sequence in which flow artifacts are possible, keep in mind:

1. What is the major direction of flow?
2. Is the part to be scanned close enough to the heart or a major vessel to require first- and second-order flow compensation?
3. Flow may not be completely removed by a flow-compensation technique because of the existence of higher orders of moments and their location. Consider adjunct compensatory measures to improve artifact suppression, such as presaturation or gating.

Flow compensation is an important artifact-suppression technique that significantly helps to minimize artifacts from flow such as CSF pulsatile flow and the slow flow from cerebral venous sinuses. This technique helps to improve image quality in anatomic regions where these two flow phenomena are most prevalent, such as the posterior fossa. The disadvantages of reduced slice thickness and longer TE are outweighed by the flow-reduction benefits of the technique.

Diagnostic accuracy in MR imaging is dependent on the selection of pulse sequences and scan parameters that will enhance image quality. When artifact-suppression techniques are incorporated into these selections, artifacts can be reduced or eliminated. The selections are chosen in a balanced manner to improve the signal-to-noise ratio, define the region of interest, and increase image contrast discrimination. Each selection will affect the resultant image in a precise and well-defined manner. The objective of the technologist/radiologist team is to chain together those pulse sequence variables that will produce an image with the best diagnostic quality in the least amount of scan time possible.

Suggested Readings

Du, LD: Flow compensation by gradient moment nulling

Elster AD: *Questions and Answers in Magnetic Resonance Imaging.* St. Louis: Mosby, 1994.

Stark DD, Bradley WG Jr.: *Magnetic Resonance Imaging.* St. Louis: Mosby, 1988.

Sweitzer JC, Kramer DM: Standard MR pulse sequences: A closer look, in Woodward P, Freimarck R: *MRI for Technologists.* New York: McGraw-Hill, 1995.

Woodward P: Assessing the interaction of image sequence parameters, in Woodward P, Freimarck R: *MRI for Technologists.* New York: McGraw-Hill, 1995.

Woodward P, Du LN: Walking with my baby or flow compensation finally explained. *Resonant Ideas,* autumn 1992, volume VI, No. 2. Continuing education newsletter for Toshiba America Medical Systems.

Young SW: *Magnetic Resonance Imaging Basic Principles,* 2d ed. New York, Raven Press, 1988.

Part *III*

Practical Imaging

---

13 Brain Imaging

The advent of magnetic resonance imaging (MRI) has resulted in a dramatic improvement in the evaluation of patients with suspected intracranial abnormalities. In order to understand what is abnormal in the human brain, it is first necessary to recognize the appearance of the normal brain.

The Normal Brain

The human brain is composed of billions of neurons, each having thousands of connections or synapses. These neurons make up most of the grey matter of the brain. The functional components of the brain reside in the gray matter. The brain also contains white matter. The white-matter connections link various parts of the brain together. These white-matter regions include the centrum semiovale, located just below the cerebral cortex; the corpus callosum, which connects the cerebral hemispheres; and the internal capsule, located between the thalamus, the caudate nucleus, and the lentiform nuclei. The nuclei of the brain and the cerebral and cerebellar cortices contain the nerve cells or neurons. These grey and white areas of the brain can be identified on MR images, and are indicated in Figs. 13-1 to 13-24.

Imaging Parameters

In general, clinical MRI of the brain employs relatively standard pulse sequences to produce images that are T1-weighted, T2-weighted, and intermediate- or proton-density-weighted. Since most of the literature on MR and virtually all MR textbooks refer to these images as they would appear on high-field-strength scanners, expectations have arisen regarding the appearance of the brain when each of these sequences is obtained. This view of the MR world has resulted in significant setbacks for lower-field-strength scanners, which may or may not produce MR brain images with the "high-field" appearance.

Regardless of the technique employed [spin echo (SE) or gradient recalled echo (GRE)], the typical MR brain scan will include a T1-weighted sequence in which fat appears white on the images and cerebral spinal fluid (CSF) is black. This has been referred to in the early MR literature as a *fat sequence* because the fat stands out as white. Clinicians have come to rely on the white fat and black CSF to inform them that this is a T1-weighted scan (see Fig. 13-25).

The T2-weighted studies, on the other hand, have been referred to as *water sequences,* since the images result in water-containing structures appearing white and fat being black (see Fig. 13-26). Many clinicians continue to rely on the appearance of fat and water to inform them of the type of scan sequence that has been obtained. This is unfortunate, since it has set a relative "standard" in MR for what a brain MRI "should look like." This has forced

Text continues on page 133.

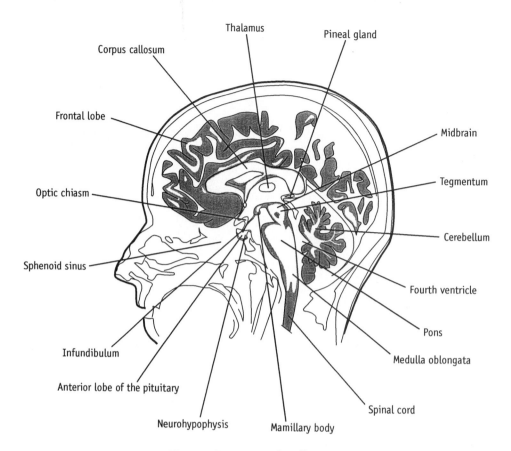

Figure 13-1 Sagittal midline MR.

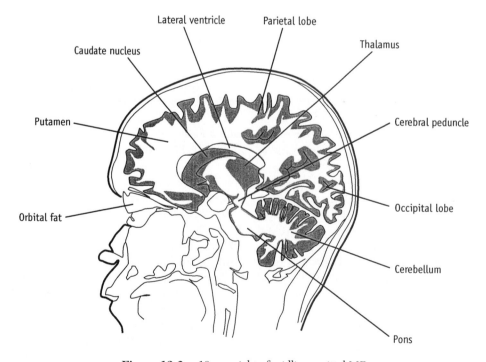

Figure 13-2 10 mm right of midline sagittal MR.

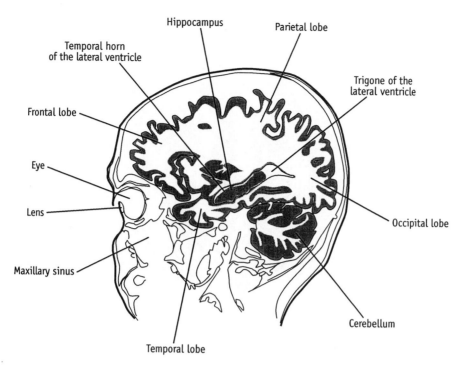

Figure 13-3 20 mm sagittal of right MR.

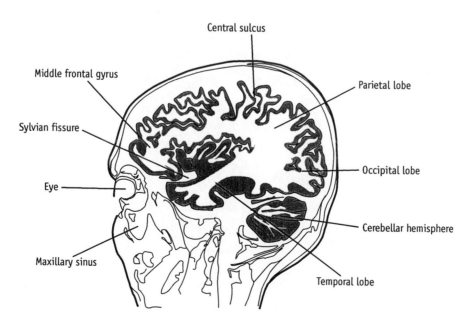

Figure 13-4 30 mm sagittal of right MR.

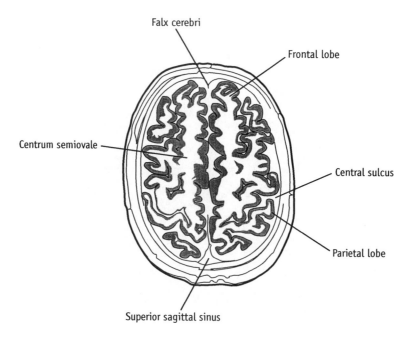

Figure 13-5   Superior axial section of MR.

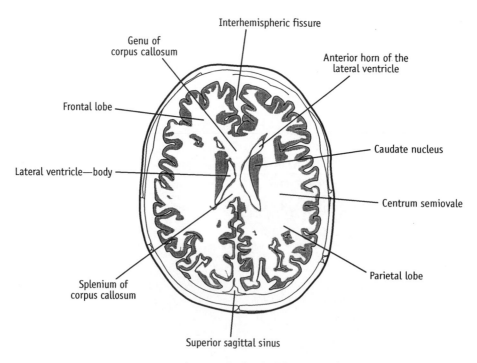

Figure 13-6   Axial MR at the level of the superior ventricles.

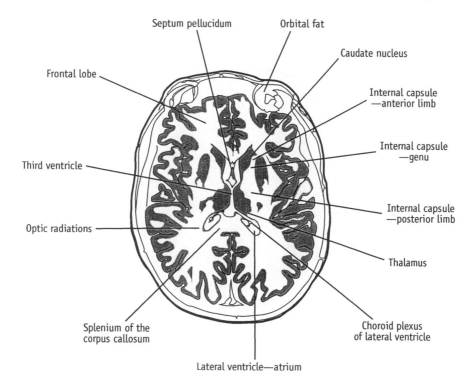

Septum pellucidum

Orbital fat

Caudate nucleus

Frontal lobe

Internal capsule
—anterior limb

Internal capsule
—genu

Third ventricle

Internal capsule
—posterior limb

Optic radiations

Thalamus

Splenium of the
corpus callosum

Choroid plexus
of lateral ventricle

Lateral ventricle—atrium

Figure 13-7   Axial MR at the level of the third and lateral ventricles.

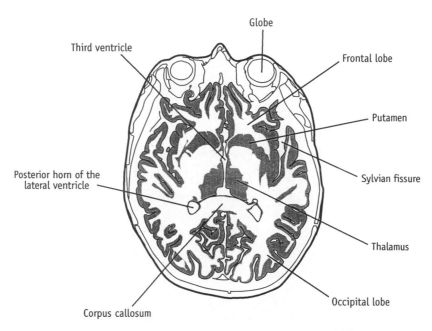

Globe

Third ventricle

Frontal lobe

Putamen

Posterior horn of the
lateral ventricle

Sylvian fissure

Thalamus

Corpus callosum

Occipital lobe

Figure 13-8   Axial MR at the level of the third ventricle and thalamus.

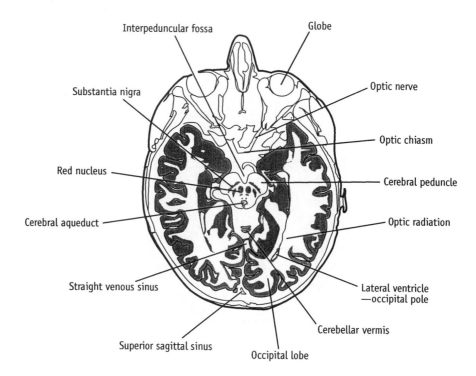

Figure 13-9   Axial MR at the level of the cerebral peduncles and aqueduct.

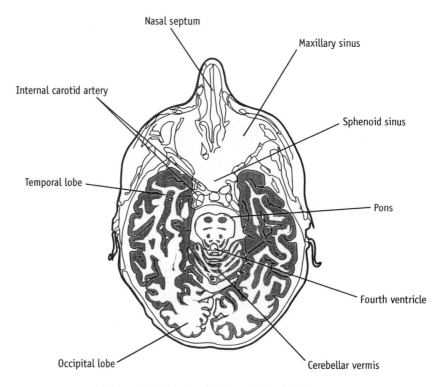

Figure 13-10   Axial MR at the level of the pons.

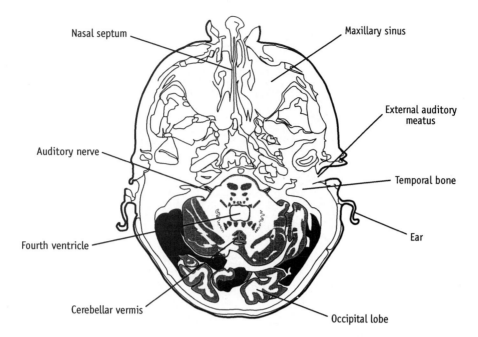

Figure 13-11   Axial MR at the level of the fourth ventricle.

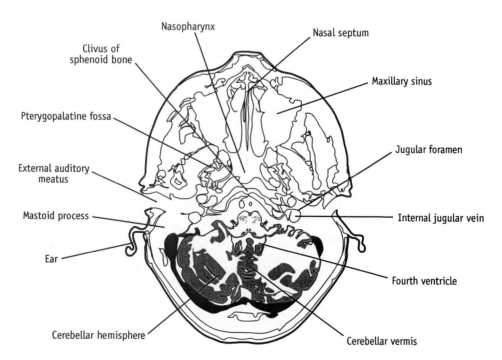

Figure 13-12   Axial MR at the level of the inferior fourth ventricle.

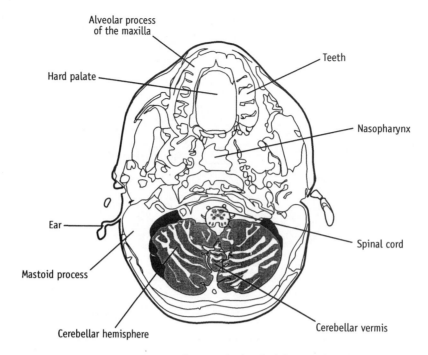

Figure 13-13   Axial MR at the level of the spinal cord.

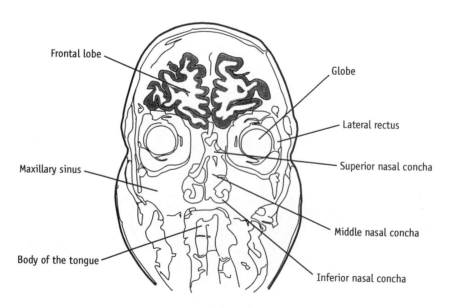

Figure 13-14   Coronal MR through the frontal lobe and orbits.

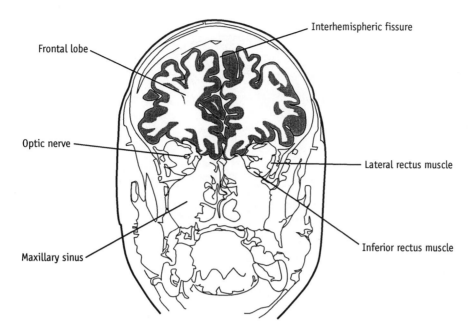

Figure 13-15   Coronal MR at the level of the orbital apex.

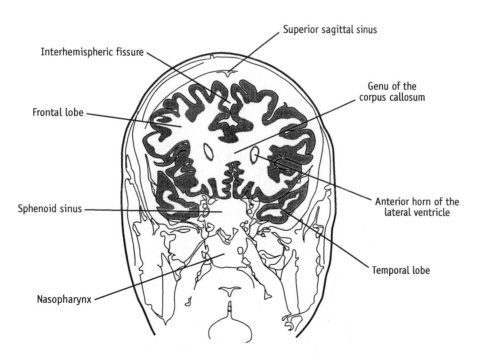

Figure 13-16   Coronal MR at the level of the anterior horns of the lateral ventricles.

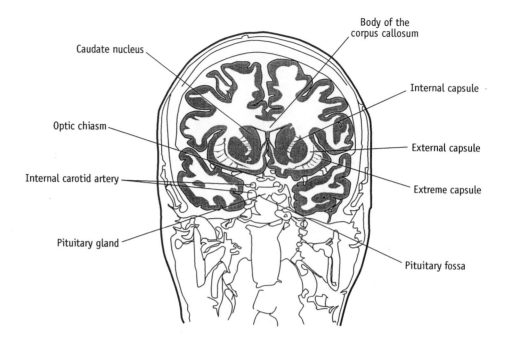

Figure 13-17 Coronal MR at the level of the optic chiasm.

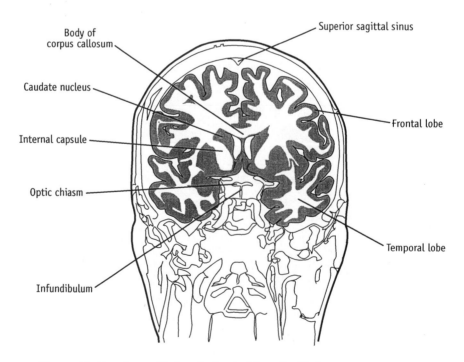

Figure 13-18 Coronal MR at the level of the infandibulum.

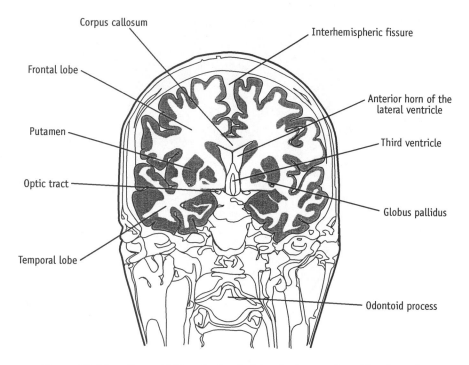

Figure 13-19   Coronal MR at the level of the third ventricle and basal ganglia.

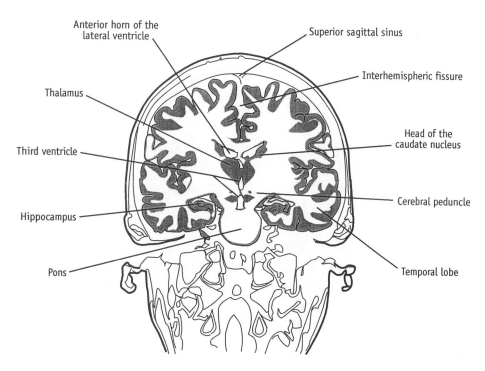

Figure 13-20   Coronal MR at the level of the third ventricle and pons.

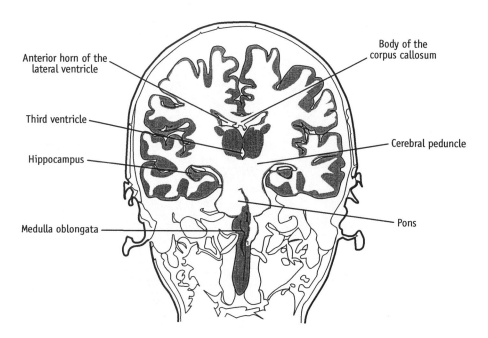

Figure 13-21 Coronal MR at the level of the medulla oblongata.

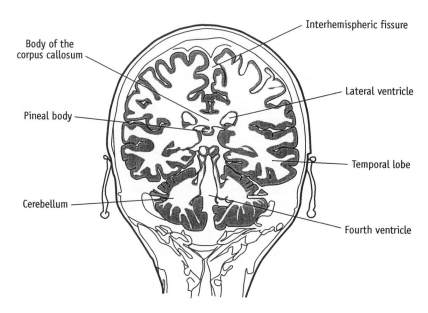

Figure 13-22 Coronal MR at the level of the fourth ventricle.

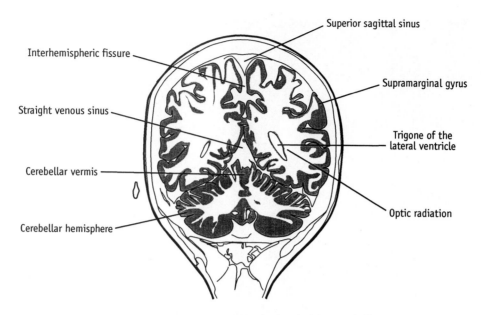

Figure 13-23   Coronal MR at the level of the cerebellum.

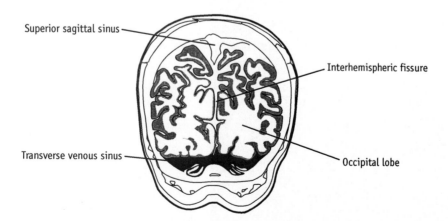

Figure 13-24   Coronal MR at the level of the occipital lobes.

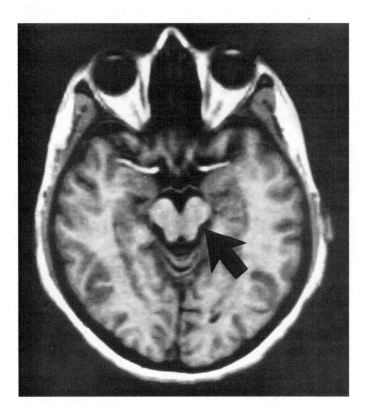

Figure 13-25   Axial T1-weighted GRE MR (TR 10, TE 4, FA 10) demonstrating the appearance of fat as white and CSF as black. Note that the orbital fat is white, outlining the optic nerves *(small arrow)*, and the CSF is black, surrounding the brainstem *(large arrow)*. Compare to Fig. 13-26.

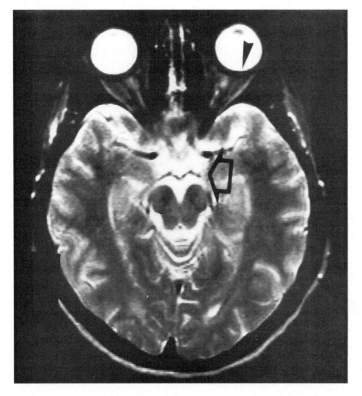

Figure 13-26   Axial T2-weighted SE MR (TR 2500, TE 90) demonstrating the appearance of water (CSF) as white and fat as black. Note that the orbital fat is black *(arrowhead)*, and the CSF surrounding the brainstem is white *(open arrow)*. Compare to Fig. 13-25.

lower-field-strength MR to attempt to look like higher-field-strength MR, and has taken away some of the advantages of lower-field-strength MR. One of the most distinctive advantages of lower-field-strength MR is the utilization of black-CSF T2-weighted sequences.

The advent of fluid attenuated inversion recovery (FLAIR) sequences has allowed for more heavily T2-weighted images with black CSF at all field strengths (Figs. 13-27A and 13-27B). At lower field strengths, it is possible to obtain relatively heavily weighted T2 sequences for which the CSF remains black using standard SE or GRE sequences. However, at higher field strengths, this requires special sequences that have only recently become available, such as FLAIR. The advantage of black-CSF T2-weighted sequences is that lesions that are white and may blend with CSF become readily identifiable (see Figs. 13-27A and 13-27B). Therefore, the "old" approach to MR images by clinicians is changing, and moving in a direction that favors the patient. That is, the imaging parameters, rather than the appearance of fat or CSF, now indicate whether the type of scan is T1, proton density, or T2 (including T2*). This will allow lower-field-strength scanners to exploit one of their main advantages, which is that black-CSF T2 techniques are more sensitive to most lesions, and consequently much easier to interpret. In some centers, black-CSF T2 techniques have entirely replaced proton-density-weighted images at all field strengths, and at lower field strengths are replacing "standard" T2 sequences as well. There is simply no advantage to white CSF in many instances other than to allow clinicians to recognize the type of scan performed. It would seem far more important for the patient that the relevant pathology be identified than that the doctor be able to tell what type of scan was done without having to "think about it."

Regardless of the appearance of CSF and fat, most lesions will appear as white on T2-weighted sequences and dark on T1-weighted sequences independent of field strength (see Figs. 13-28 and 13-29). This is generally true of all types of pathology. However, the use of intravenous contrast agents may allow for the identification of abnormalities that would have gone undetected by noncontrast methods.

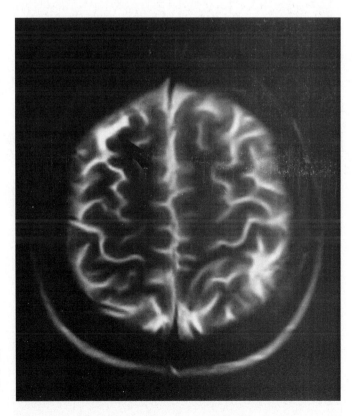

Figure 13-27A Axial T2-weighted SE MR (TR 3000, TE 120) demonstrating the appearance of water (CSF) as white. Note how the lesion (*arrow*) is similar in signal intensity to the surrounding CSF. Compare to Fig. 13-27B.

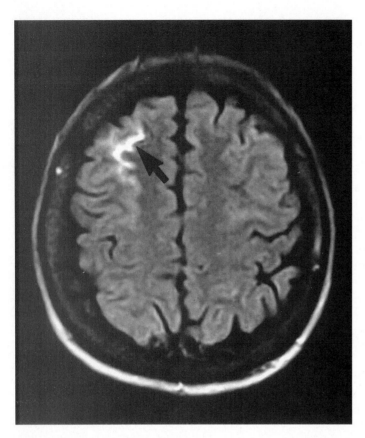

Figure 13-27B Axial T2-weighted MR with black CSF (FLAIR, TI 1600, TR 4750, TE 120). Compare to Fig. 13-27A and note the obvious right frontal lesion *(arrow)* that is difficult to see when the CSF is white.

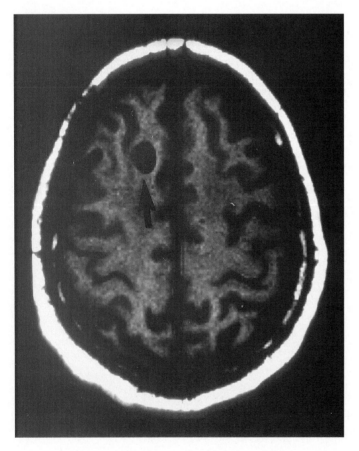

Figure 13-28 Cystic lesion on axial T1-weighted SE MR (TR 600, TE 15), demonstrating low signal intensity within the lesion *(arrow)*. Compare to Fig. 13-29.

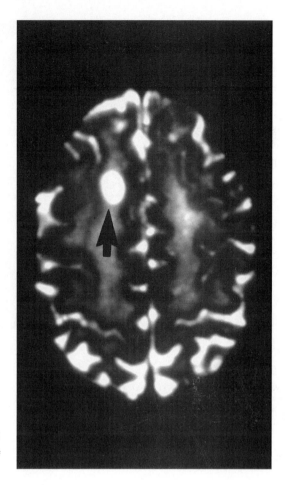

Figure 13-29 Cystic lesion on axial T2-weighted SE MR (TR 2500, TE 90), demonstrating high signal intensity within the lesion *(arrow)*. Compare to Fig. 13-28.

Contrast Agents

Typically, intravenous contrast agents are given in MR in order to enhance areas of abnormality that might otherwise be difficult or impossible to detect. Normal structures such as the dural sinuses, pituitary gland and stalk, and orbital muscles will also be enhanced (Figs. 13-30*A* and 13-30*B*). The most commonly used intravenous contrast agent in MR is currently gadolinium diethylenetriamine pentaacetic acid (Gd-DTPA, gadopentetate dimeglumine). This is a relatively nontoxic paramagnetic agent that produces enhancement by altering the local magnetic environment. The contrast agent is not observed directly, but rather in the magnetic effect on nearby hydrogen nuclei. The agent acts as a relaxation center for other nuclei in the local microenvironment and thereby shortens the magnetic relaxation times of the surrounding hydrogen nuclei. Standard dosages range from 0.1 to 0.3 mmol/kg. Such contrast agents are effective secondary to a breakdown in the blood-brain barrier or as a result of increased vascularity in pathologic tissue. The normal blood-brain barrier prevents the contrast agent from entering the brain, but when this barrier is disrupted by a disease process, the contrast agent can leak into the abnormal tissue, allowing the enhancement to occur. MRI contrast is approximately 20 times greater than CT contrast, and much safer. Therefore, MRI contrast is often considered the procedure of choice in the evaluation of primary and secondary (metastatic) brain tumors (Figs. 13-31*A*, 13-31*B*, and 13-31*C*).

MR in Brain Disorders

MR is utilized clinically for virtually every type of brain pathology. The value of a normal MR brain examination is not to be underestimated, since this may drastically alter

Text continues on page 138.

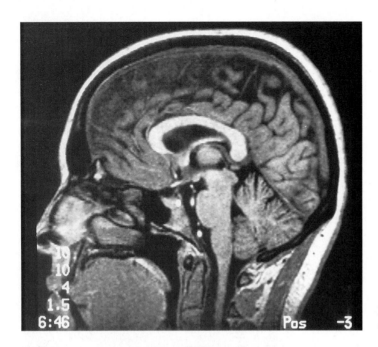

Figure 13-30A Normal sagittal T1-weighted GRE MR (TR 10, TE 4, FA 10). Compare to Fig. 13-30*B*.

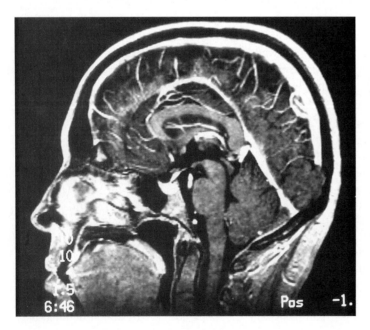

Figure 13-30B Normal contrast-enhanced sagittal T1-weighted GRE MR (TR 10, TE 4, FA 10) performed following the administration of 0.1 mmol of Gd-DTPA. Compare to Fig. 13-30*A* and note the enhancement of the dural sinuses and the pituitary gland and stalk.

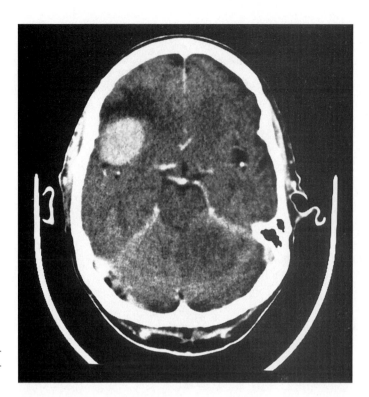

Figure 13-31A Axial contrast-enhanced CT scan demonstrating abnormal enhancement in a brain neoplasm. Compare to Figs. 13-31B and 13-31C.

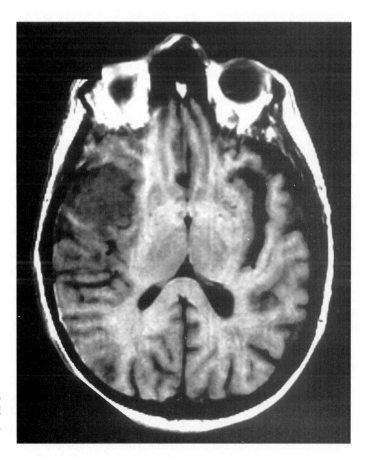

Figure 13-31B Axial T1-weighted SE MR (TR 700, TE 15) without contrast enhancement, demonstrating low signal intensity within the brain tumor. Compare to Figs. 13-31A and 13-31C.

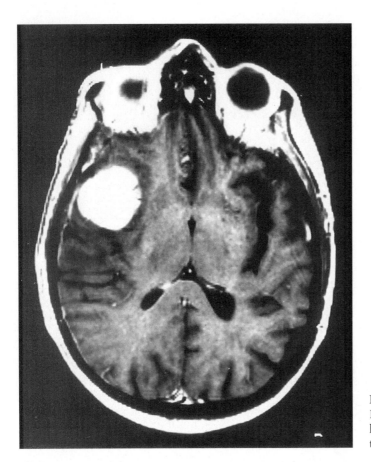

Figure 13-31C Axial contrast-enhanced T1-weighted SE MR (TR 700, TE 15), demonstrating abnormal contrast enhancement seen as very high signal intensity within the brain tumor. Compare to Figs. 13-31A and 13-31B.

the planned treatment approach, not to mention the relief it gives to the patient and the referring physician. In fact, the normal brain MR may be one of the most cost-effective studies in all of medicine. Not only does it preclude most forms of significant brain pathology, but it also expedites the patient's exit from the most expensive area of the health care system. However, much more attention is given to the abnormal brain MR, and it is important for the MR technologist to be able to identify at least the most severely abnormal scans. This is important from the standpoint of recognizing before the patient leaves the scanner that additional sequences may be required, and also to protect the patient from leaving the health care environment with a dangerous brain abnormality.

Neoplasms

Approximately 40,000 patients in the United States are identified annually as having new brain tumors, and most

of these receive an MR examination of the brain. The recognizable characteristics of a neoplasm on MR studies of the brain include mass effect, edema, hemorrhage, and contrast enhancement. The typical features of a brain neoplasm are demonstrated in Figs. 13-32A, 13-32B, and 13-32C. Brain tumors are classified as being benign or malignant pathologically, but because of the nature of the brain, these classifications may not apply. Even the most "benign" tumor may be devastatingly incapacitating or even fatal if it is located in a vital part of the brain. Although many brain tumors continue to be refractory to treatment, the number of neoplasms that can be effectively treated is increasing (see Figs. 13-33A and 13-33B).

Brain tumors are frequently viewed on MR as being *intraaxial,* that is, within the brain substance, or *extraaxial,* meaning outside the brain substance. Extraaxial neoplasms are more commonly benign, and in general easier to resect surgically (see Figs. 13-33A and 13-33B). Malignant tumors are most often intraaxial, and frequently extend far into the brain beyond the appearance on MR (see

Text continues on page 142.

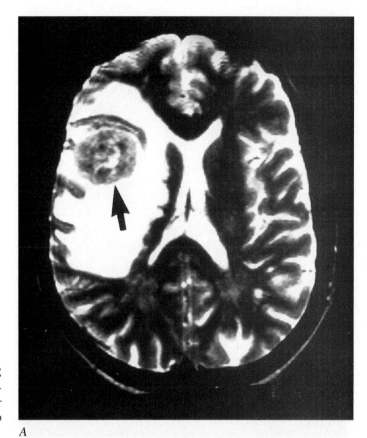

Figure 13-32A Axial T2-weighted SE MR (TR 2700, TE 90), demonstrating high signal from edema around the tumor *(white area containing the arrow)* and relatively lower signal intensity within the brain tumor *(arrow)*. Compare to Figs. 13-32B and 13-32C.

A

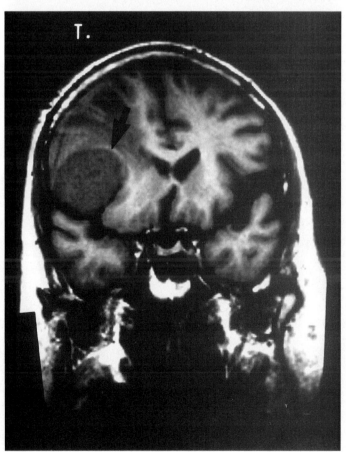

Figure 13-32B Coronal T1-weighted SE MR (TR 700, TE 15) without contrast enhancement, demonstrating low signal intensity within the edema surrounding the brain tumor *(dark area containing the arrow)* and relatively higher signal intensity within the brain tumor *(arrow)*. Compare to Figs. 13-32A and 13-32C.

B

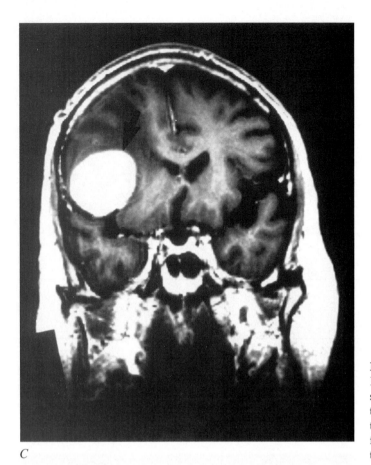

C

Figure 13-32 *(Continued)   C*. Coronal T1-weighted SE MR (TR 700, TE 15) with contrast enhancement, demonstrating low signal intensity within the edema surrounding the brain tumor *(dark area containing the arrow)* and extremely high signal intensity within the brain tumor *(arrow)* following the administration of intravenous Gd-DTPA contrast. Compare to Figs. 13-32*A* and 13-32*B*.

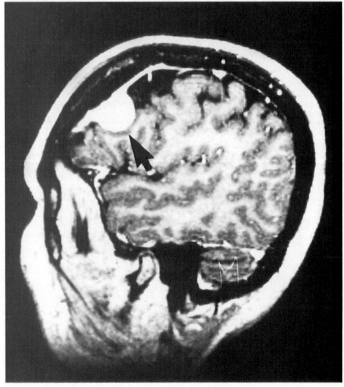

A

Figure 13-33   *A*. Sagittal T1-weighted GRE MR (TR 10, TE 4, FA 10) with contrast enhancement, demonstrating high signal intensity within a meningioma *(arrow)*. Compare to Fig. 13-33*B*.

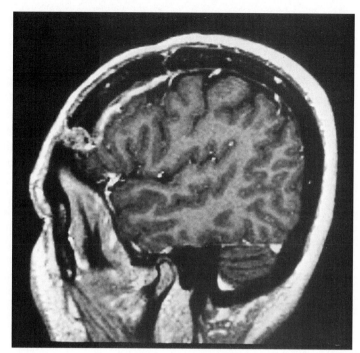

Figure 13-33 *(Continued)* *B*. Sagittal T1-weighted GRE MR (TR 10, TE 4, FA 10) with contrast enhancement demonstrating complete removal of this benign brain tumor. Compare to Fig. 13-33*A*.

B

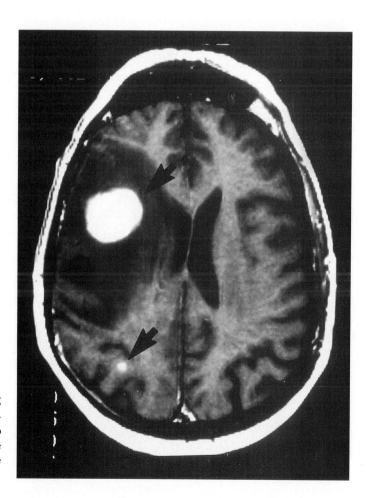

Figure 13-34 Axial contrast-enhanced T1-weighted SE MR (TR 700, TE 15), demonstrating abnormal contrast enhancement seen as very high signal intensity within two metastatic breast cancer foci to the brain *(arrows)*. Note the difference in size of these two lesions that are both from the same primary tumor.

Fig. 13-32). This makes surgical cure difficult, and recurrence common. These tumors include metastatic cancer from other organ systems.

Metastatic cancer, most commonly arising from primary neoplasms of the lung and breast, represents approximately 25 percent of all brain tumors (see Fig. 13-34). In addition, metastatic brain tumors may arise from the gastrointestinal tract, the genitourinary tract, and melanoma. Hemorrhage is common in metastatic tumors, and most enhance with contrast. It is important to remember that a history of steroid therapy can block contrast enhancement, and a double or triple dose of contrast may be required to demonstrate brain tumors in patients on steroids. For the MR technologist, one quick way to positive fame is to remind the physician that a patient about to receive intravenous contrast is on steroid therapy. The resulting increase in contrast may drastically alter the patient's subsequent care (see Figs. 13-35A and 13-35B).

Infections

Brain infections are becoming one of the more common indications for brain imaging, and it is important for the MR technologist to remember that many of these infections may be contagious. Universal precautions to protect against the spread of disease are indicated in all patients, but the alert technologist will be particularly careful when dealing with a known or potentially infected patient.

Infection of the brain may be the result of extension of infectious conditions in the sinuses, ear, orbit, or superficial soft tissues. In addition, the infection can be carried via the bloodstream from various parts of the body. Regardless of the nature of the brain infection, these are some of the most urgent and important scans that the MR technologist will perform. This is because many of these conditions respond rapidly to treatment. In instances of

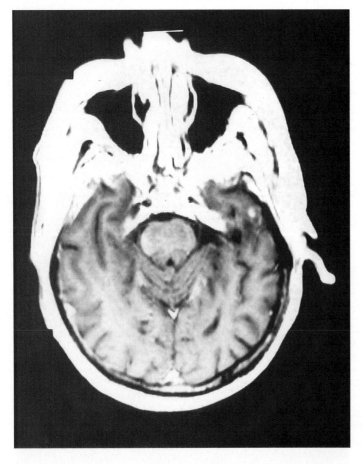

Figure 13-35A Axial contrast-enhanced T1-weighted SE MR (TR 600, TE 15), demonstrating no abnormal contrast enhancement. The patient was scanned again on the same day using double-dose contrast after the technologist learned that the patient was on steroids.

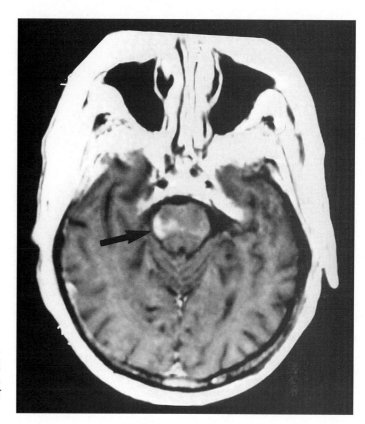

Figure 13-35B Axial *double-dose* contrast-enhanced T1-weighted SE MR (TR 600, TE 15), demonstrating abnormal contrast enhancement, seen as high signal intensity within the brainstem *(arrow)*. Note the difference in the degree of enhancement compared to Fig. 13-35A.

brain infection, early treatment may mean the difference between the patient's being normal, being severely incapacitated, or dying (see Figs. 13-36A and 13-36B).

Vascular Disease

Cerebrovascular disease represents the third leading cause of death in the United States. Most of this cerebrovascular disease affects individuals over the age of 55, and is related to atherosclerotic disease. Patients with cerebrovascular disorders who present for MR will commonly be suffering from one of three conditions: (1) a transient ischemic attack (TIA), in which there is a temporary neurological deficit that clears in less than 24 h, (2) a reversible ischemic neurologic deficit (RIND), during which the patient suffers a neurologic deficit of longer than 24 h duration, but which still clears, or (3) a cerebrovascular accident (CVA), or completed stroke, from

which the patient does not entirely recover lost neurologic function. A fourth condition for which MR, and particularly MRA (magnetic resonance angiography), may be used is a "stroke in progress." This is a medical emergency, and is now commonly treated in a manner similar to a heart attack. In fact, the term *brain attack* has been coined to convey the urgency of this condition. The technologist who is confronted with a patient who is having a brain attack must move quickly and decisively in all regards. In this circumstance, literally every second counts. When treatment is early and effectively rendered, it has been possible to entirely reverse strokes that would have otherwise left the patient paralyzed.

The MR scan in TIA or RIND is usually normal or minimally abnormal. However, when a patient with a stroke or stroke in progress (brain attack) is scanned by MR, the examination will frequently be very abnormal. The MR will also be abnormal long before the CT shows a problem, and therefore MR is being used increasingly in the early evaluation of patients suspected of having a stroke. In early stroke, the examination will demonstrate edema and mass effect, with the abnormalities being most prevalent on T2-weighted sequences (see Fig. 13-37).

Text continues on page 146.

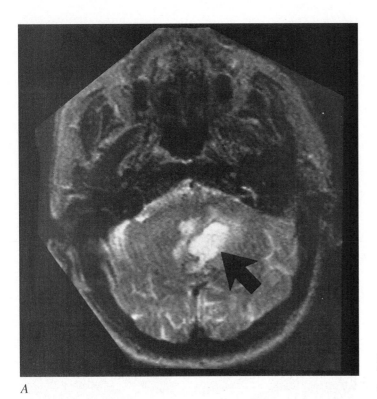

A

Figure 13-36A Axial T2-weighted SE MR (TR 2500, TE 90), demonstrating high signal from an abscess *(arrow)*. Compare to Fig. 13-36B.

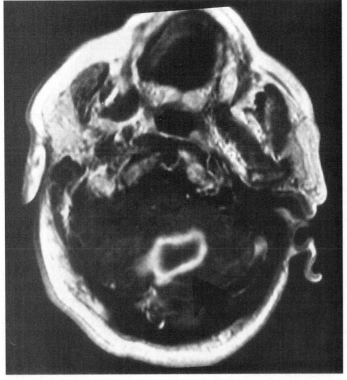

B

Figure 13-36B Axial contrast-enhanced T1-weighted SE MR (TR 600, TE 15), demonstrating abnormal contrast enhancement, seen as a rim of high signal intensity within the cerebellum *(arrow)*. Compare the appearance of this abscess to Fig. 13-36A.

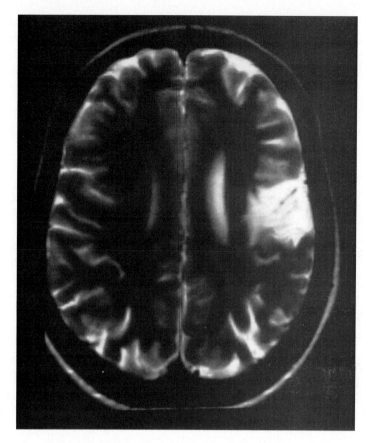

Figure 13-37 Axial T2-weighted SE MR (TR 3500, TE 93), demonstrating high signal from a recent stroke. Compare to Fig. 13-38.

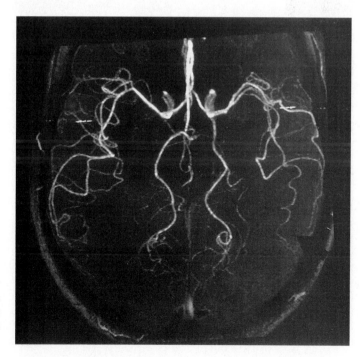

Figure 13-38 Maximum intensity projection (MIP) magnetization transfer (MT) MRA (TR 43, TE 8, FA 20), demonstrating loss of normal cerebral vasculature in the left middle cerebral artery territory *(arrow)*. Compare to the blood vessels of the opposite side and Fig. 13-37.

MRA may be particularly beneficial in identifying the occluded blood vessel (see Fig. 13-38). As the stroke evolves or ages, the abnormality will appear more or less similar to CSF, and local brain atrophy will ultimately occur (see Fig. 13-39). The cause of the loss of brain substance is often an abnormality at the carotid bifurcation in the neck, and MRA may demonstrate the atherosclerotic disease of the carotid artery quite well (see Figs. 13-40A and 13-40B). MR contrast enhancement may improve the detection, dating, and grading of cerebral infarction (stroke) (see Figs. 13-41A and 13-41B).

Additional forms of cerebrovascular disease that may be identified by MR include aneurysms and arteriovenous malformation. MRA may improve the definition of these lesions, and MRA is commonly performed for the evaluation or exclusion of these types of disorders. In addition, magnetic resonance venography (MRV) may assist in demonstrating the markedly abnormal veins that often accompany vascular disorders in the brain (see Fig. 13-42).

Head Trauma

Traumatic brain injury is one of the most common types of insult in the United States, with more than 2 million cases each year. MR has been shown to be far more effective in the evaluation of traumatic brain injury than CT,

and MR is becoming increasingly utilized for this injury (see Figs. 13-43A and 13-43B). The types of lesions that can be better identified by MR than by CT include contusions, shearing injury of the white matter, subdural hematomas, epidural hematomas, and anoxic injury.

Hemorrhage

Perhaps the most difficult area to understand in all of MR imaging of the brain is the appearance of hemorrhage. Many published studies have addressed the appearance of blood on MR, and there is as much disagreement as there is agreement on this topic. This is to a large extent due to the fact that field strength has been ignored when hemorrhage on MR is considered. When the field strength of the scanner is included, a common pattern in the appearance of intraparenchymal hemorrhage is identifiable.

In the hyperacute stage of hemorrhage (bleeding that is less than 24 h in age), T1- and T2-weighted images will show hyperintensity. T1 will be much more hyperintense as the field strength decreases, and T2 will rapidly lose intensity as the field strength increases. In other words, look for hyperacute blood to be white on T1 at low field strength and white on T2 at both high and low field strengths, but not for long at higher field strengths (see Figs. 13-44A and 13-44B).

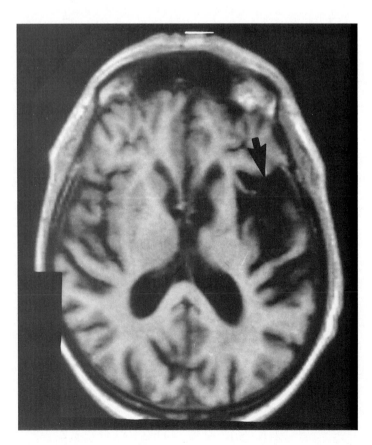

Figure 13-39 Axial T1-weighted GRE MR (TR 10, TE 4, FA 10), demonstrating an area of CSF signal intensity *(arrow)* from an old stroke.

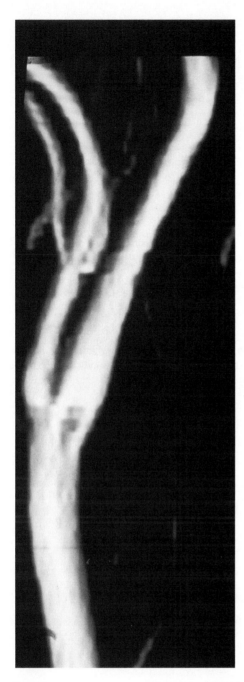

Figure 13-40A Maximum intensity projection (MIP) magnetization transfer (MT) MRA (TR 30, TE 9, FA 60), demonstrating a normal carotid bifurcation. Compare to the abnormal blood vessels in Fig. 13-40B.

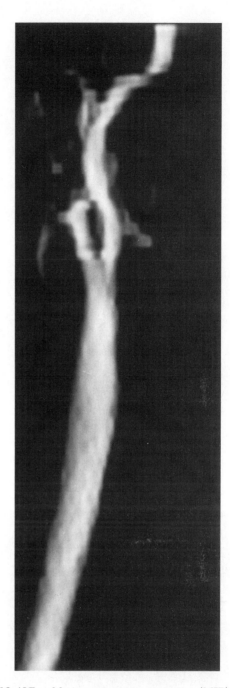

Figure 13-40B Maximum intensity projection (MIP) magnetization transfer (MT) MRA (TR 30, TE 9, FA 60), demonstrating an abnormal carotid bifurcation resulting from atherosclerotic disease. Compare to the normal blood vessels in Fig. 13-40A.

As blood ages, it becomes acute (1 day to 1 week) and loses intensity on both T1 and T2 sequences at all field strengths. However, it will become darker more rapidly at higher field strengths on both T1- and particularly T2-weighted sequences. This is due to a combination of clot retraction and deoxyhemoglobin formation as well as red blood cell settling and packing (see Figs. 13-45A and 13-45B).

As blood continues to age, it becomes subacute (2 weeks to 1 month) and goes through several phases. Initially, intracellular methemoglobin begins to form, and T1-weighted sequences show the blood as white (increased signal intensity or hyperintensity), while T2 sequences show decreased signal continually (see Figs. 13-46A and 13-46B). Next, the methemoglobin becomes extracellular as the red blood cells lyse, and then

Text continues on page 153.

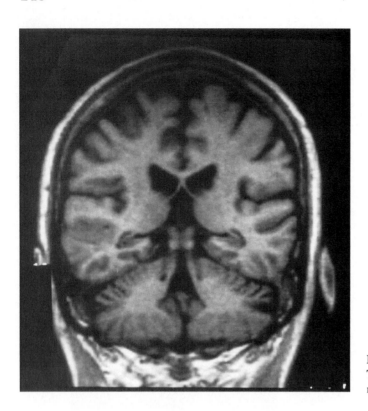

Figure 13-41A Coronal T1-weighted GRE MR (TR 10, TE 4, FA 10) without contrast, demonstrating minimal abnormality. Compare to Fig. 13-41*B*.

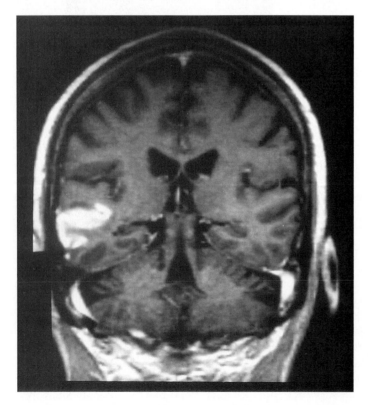

Figure 13-41B Coronal T1-weighted GRE MR (TR 10, TE 4, FA 10) with abnormal contrast enhancement, demonstrated as high signal intensity within an area of recent cerebral infarction (stroke).

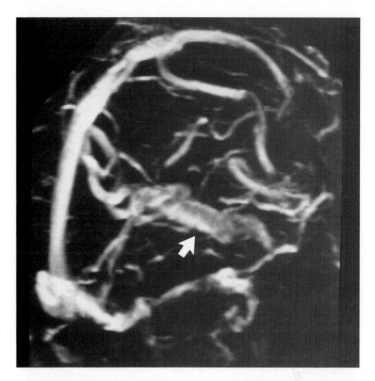

Figure 13-42 Maximum intensity projection (MIP) MRV (TR 32, TE 10, FA 50), demonstrating a markedly abnormal and enlarged draining vein in a patient with a cerebral arterovenous malformation.

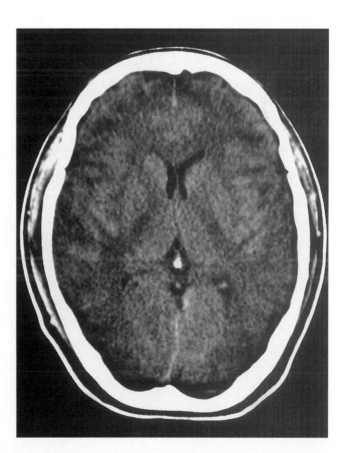

Figure 13-43A Axial CT of the head following trauma, demonstrating no significant abnormality. Compare to Fig. 13-43B.

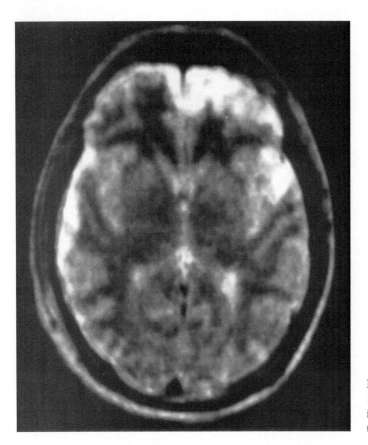

Figure 13-43B Axial T2-weighted SE MR (TR 2000, TE 105), demonstrating multiple areas of abnormally high signal in regions of brain injury. Compare to Fig. 13-43A and note the improved sensitivity of MR over CT in head trauma.

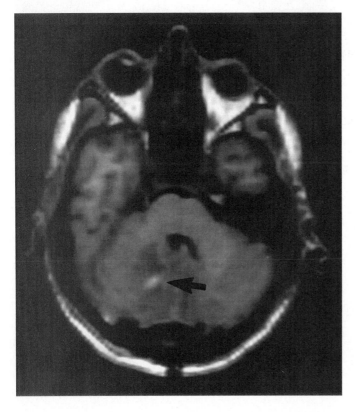

Figure 13-44A Axial T1-weighted GRE MR (TR 30, TE 10, FA 35), with increased signal intensity in an area of hyperacute hemorrhage (*arrow*). Compare to Fig. 13-44B.

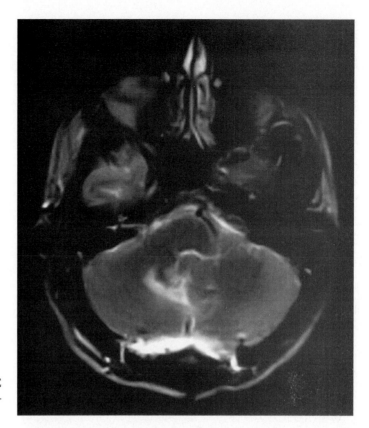

Figure 13-44*B* Axial T2-weighted SE MR (TR 2900, TE 120), demonstrating high signal in an area of hyperacute hemorrhage. Compare to Fig. 13-44*A*.

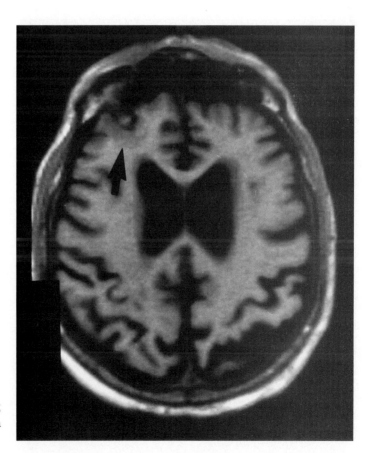

Figure 13-45*A* Axial T1-weighted GRE MR (TR 10, TE 4, FA 10), with slightly decreased signal intensity in an area of acute hemorrhage. Compare to Fig. 13-45*B*.

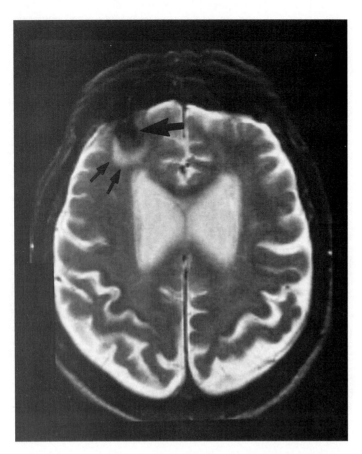

Figure 13-45B Axial T2-weighted SE MR (TR 2500, TE 90), demonstrating high signal from edema *(small arrows)* and decreased signal *(large arrow)* from acute hemorrhage (5 days). Note how much the central signal *(large arrow)* has decreased compared to the T1 image in Fig. 13-45A.

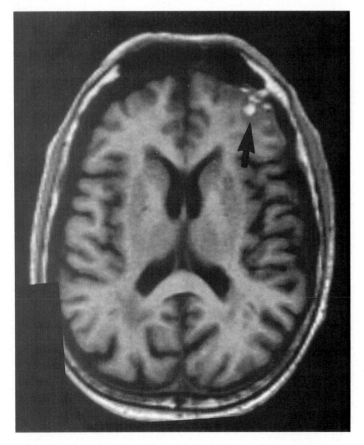

Figure 13-46A Axial T1-weighted GRE MR (TR 10, TE 4, FA 10) with increased signal intensity in an area of subacute hemorrhage as a result of intracellular methemoglobin. Compare to Figs. 13-45A and 13-46B.

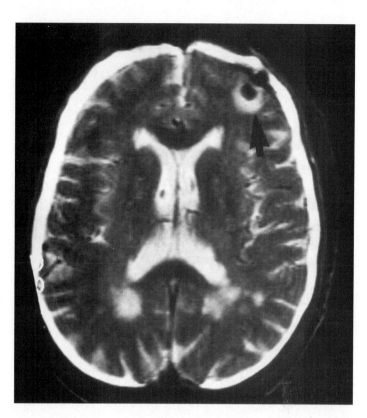

Figure 13-46B   Axial T2-weighted SE MR (TR 2500, TE 90), demonstrating high signal from edema and decreased signal from subacute hemorrhage *(arrow)*. Note how the central signal *(arrow)* remains decreased compared to the increased signal on the T1 image in Fig. 13-46A in this hemorrhage that is now 2 weeks old. Also present are bilateral subdural hygromas (white rim around the brain) from old trauma. Compare this to Fig. 13-46A, where this rim is dark.

blood becomes hyperintense (white) on T2 sequences also.

When blood becomes more than a month old, it is generally referred to as chronic. At this time, blood will remain hyperintense (white) on both T1- and T2-weighted sequences until it is replaced by CSF (see Figs. 13-47A and 13-47B). Then it will usually be hyperintense (white) on T2 and hypointense (black) on T1.

The changes that blood goes through on MR are summarized in Fig. 13-48. Figure 13-49 illustrates the effect of field strength on the appearance of blood over time. Essentially, blood goes through the exact same changes at all field strengths, but the time course is more rapid at lower field strengths. Although many patients with intracranial hemorrhage may be hard for the technologist to manage, even scans with significant motion artifact may be diagnostic (see Figs. 13-47A and 13-47B).

White Matter Disease

Basically, white matter disease of the brain is well evaluated only by MR. There is no other technique that can ri-

val MR in studying white matter disease. Therefore, MR is indicated whenever white matter disease of the brain is suspected. Traditionally, white matter disease has been classified as either demyelinating or dysmyelinating. Dysmyelinating disease refers to a group of conditions in which there is a lack of normal myelin (white matter) formation in the brain. Examples of these types of conditions include metachromatic leukodystrophy, Krabbe's disease (globoid cell leukodystrophy), Canavan's disease (spongiform leukodystrophy), Alexander's disease (fibrinoid leukodystrophy), and adrenal leukodystrophy. They all have in common a lack or delay in the formation of normal white matter, resulting in severe neurologic abnormalities and/or early death (see Fig. 13-50).

Demyelinating conditions are thought to be diseases in which there is a loss of normally formed myelin, in contrast to the dysmyelinating diseases, where there was no normal myelin formed. Although there are many disorders that can ultimately result in the loss of normally formed myelin, the most common condition considered when demyelination is present is multiple sclerosis (MS). These patients have highly variable forms of clinical presentation, which is more or less the hallmark of this dis-

Text continues on page 157.

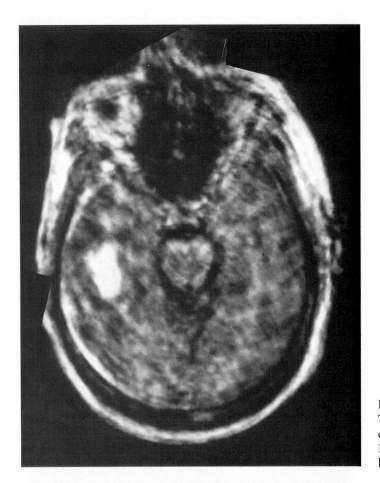

Figure 13-47A Axial T1-weighted GRE MR (TR 10, TE 4, FA 10) with increased signal intensity in an area of chronic (1 month) hemorrhage. Compare to Fig. 13-47*B*. Note that there is image degradation due to patient motion; however, the hemorrhage remains obvious.

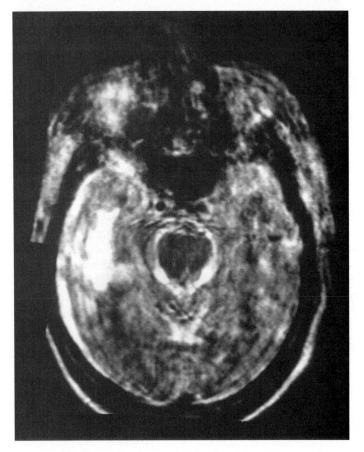

Figure 13-47B Axial T2-weighted SE MR (TR 2500, TE 90), demonstrating high signal from chronic hemorrhage. Compare to the T1 image in Fig. 13-47*A*.

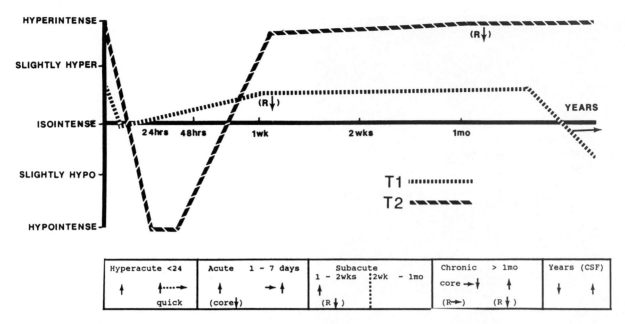

Figure 13-48   Graph demonstrating the temporal pattern of hemorrhage at low field strength (0.02 T). (*Arrows indicate increased, decreased, or isointensity.*) (After Chaney et al., with permission.)

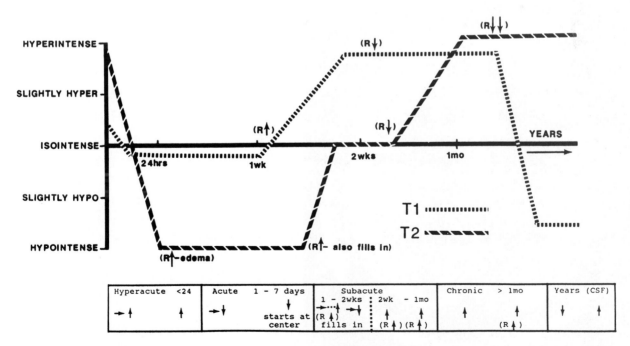

Figure 13-49   Graph demonstrating the temporal pattern of hemorrhage at high field strength (1.5 T). (*Arrows indicate increased, decreased, or isointensity.*) (After Chaney et al, with permission.)

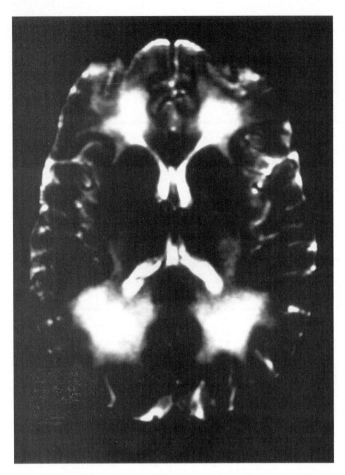

Figure 13-50 Axial T2-weighted SE MR (TR 2500, TE 90), demonstrating abnormally high signal intensity in the white matter from metachromatic leukodystrophy.

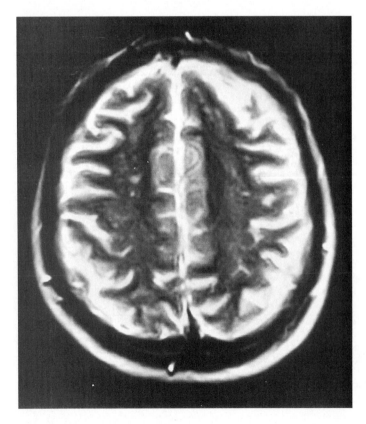

Figure 13-51A Axial T2-weighted SE MR (TR 2900, TE 120), demonstrating no definite abnormal signal intensity.

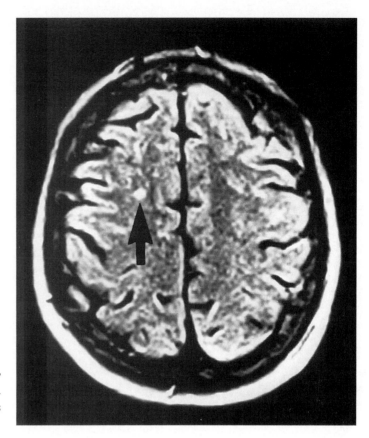

Figure 13-51B   Axial T2-weighted MR with black CSF (FLAIR, TI 1600, TR 4750, TE 120). Compare to Fig. 13-51A and note the obvious right frontal lesion *(arrow)* that is difficult to see on standard T2 sequencing

ease. It is the broad variety of neurologic symptoms occurring at different times that often leads to a suspicion of MS. The MR appearance is that of multiple periventricular hyperintense lesions on T2-weighted sequences, and this is the type of scan in which black-CSF techniques can be quite important. Since the CSF is white on routine high-field-strength T2 methods, and the lesions are also white on T2, early disease can be missed. However, with black-CSF techniques, the lesions remain white but are now against a black CSF signal that makes missing the lesions nearly impossible (see Fig. 13-51B).

always necessary, but in the case of these patients it cannot be overemphasized. Even the patient with a normal brain MR is probably very worried about the results of the scan, and in some instances the patient may still have a functional brain abnormality that MR is unable to diagnose.

A brain MR may be just another scan in a long day's work to the MR technologist, but to the patient it is probably one of the most frightening events of his or her life, regardless of the outcome. The MR technologist is in a position to be kind, caring, compassionate, and understanding. With each scan performed, the MR technologist has the opportunity to make a lasting difference in a patient's life.

Summary

The MR technologist plays an important role in the evaluation of patients suspected of having a brain disorder. Often these patients have the most to fear and the least to look forward to in life. A sensitive and caring approach is

Suggested Readings

Atlas SW (ed.): *Magnetic Resonance Imaging of the Brain and Spine*. New York: Raven Press, 1991.

Chaney RK, Taber KH, Orrison WW Jr., Hayman LA: Magnetic resonance imaging of intracerebral hemorrhage at different field strengths: A review of reported intraparenchymal signal intensities. *Neuroimaging Clinics of North America* 2(1): 25–51, 1992.

Latchaw RE (ed.): *MR and CT Imaging of the Head, Neck, and Spine,* Vols. 1 and 2, 2d ed. St. Louis: Mosby-Year Book, 1991.

Orrison WW Jr.: *Introduction to Neuroimaging.* Boston: Little, Brown, 1989.

Ramsey RG: *Neuroradiology,* 3d ed. Philadelphia: W. B. Saunders, 1994.

14

Cervical Spine Imaging

MR imaging of the cervical spine is performed for a variety of clinical reasons, including the evaluation of degenerative disease, trauma, primary neoplasms, metastatic change, and disorders of the spinal cord. The cervical spine is somewhat unique in that the vertebral bodies are smaller than those of the thoracic and lumbar spine, and of course this part of the spine articulates with the base of the skull. The cervical articulating processes of the vertebral column are larger and more lateral than those in the remainder of the spine. They are termed *lateral masses* at the level of C1 because of their size.

The Normal Cervical Spine

The appearance of the normal cervical spine on MR is shown in Figs. 14-1, 14-2, and 14-3. In general, the sagittal MR images of the cervical spine will best demonstrate the spinal cord, the intervertebral discs, the soft tissues of the neck, and the inferior aspect of the posterior cranial fossa. On T1-weighted sequences, the vertebral bodies will appear similar in intensity to the vertebral discs, or be slightly hyperintense to the adjacent disc. The CSF within the spinal canal is dark on T1-weighted sequences, with the spinal cord of relatively higher signal intensity. The neural foramina are not well visualized on the sagittal examination, and axial images provide a significantly better view of these structures (see Fig. 14-3). On T2-weighted (SE or GRE) sequences, the CSF is hyperintense (white), so that the spinal cord is of comparably lower signal intensity. The intervertebral discs will normally be of increased signal intensity as well, although less so than in the lumbar spine (see Fig. 14-2). GRE sequences may be preferred, since these sequences provide for improved definition of disc and bone as well as adjacent ligaments (see Fig. 14-3). Axial T2-weighted images will show the disc to be of relatively high signal, as is the CSF. Therefore, the bone and ligaments will stand out as black against this white background. In addition, the spinal cord and nerve roots will appear darker than the surrounding CSF, and the neural foramina will be well visualized as a result of the hyperintense CSF (see Fig. 14-3).

Diseases of the Cervical Spine

Disease processes that can affect the cervical spine include degenerative disorders, infections, neoplasms, trauma, demyelinating diseases, vascular malformations, ischemia, and other less common conditions such as syringomyelia. By far the most frequently encountered abnormal condition in routine clinical practice is degenerative disease. The degenerative process may involve any part of the cervical spine, and usually predominantly affects the vertebral bodies, the intervertebral discs, and the neuronal foramina.

Degenerative disease may lead to misalignment, with one vertebral body offset relative to the next (see Fig. 14-4). This is generally referred to as subluxation, and may be associated with significant narrowing of the spinal canal. Narrowing of the cervical spinal canal as a result of degenerative disease is not at all uncommon, and when it involves compression of the spinal cord, the clinical symptoms can be quite severe. Spinal cord compression can lead to weakness, spasticity, and loss of normal sensation (see Fig. 14-5). Narrowing of the neural foramina is another sequela of degenerative disease of the cervical spine, and this can also lead to neurological impairment (see Fig. 14-6). Another commonly encountered condition that may be related to degenerative disease or trauma is the protruding or herniated intervertebral disc. This condition can be severe enough to lead to cord compression, and there is often an associated narrowing of the neural foramen on the involved side, with nerve root compromise (see Fig. 14-7).

As was mentioned previously, the cervical spine is unique in that it articulates with the base of the skull. Therefore, disease conditions that affect the craniocervical junction are often identified on MR studies of the cervical spine. The anatomy of this region is such that the brain is contiguous with the spinal cord, and this area is referred to as the cervicomedullary junction.

This level of the central nervous system (CNS) is of particular clinical importance, since the control of vital life functions such as cardiac and respiratory activity is located here. In addition, disease processes that affect this

159

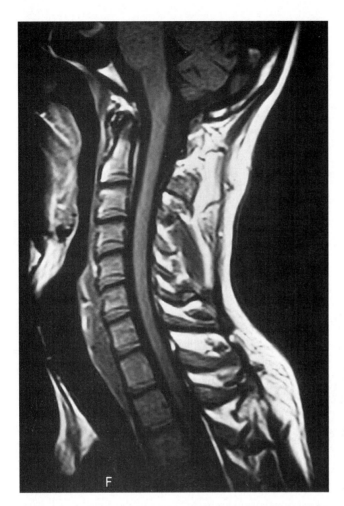

Figure 14-1   Sagittal SE T1-weighted MR (TR 500, TE 16) demonstrating the normal appearance of the cervical spine. Note that the spinal cord is seen as a relatively higher signal against the darker surrounding CSF. Compare to Fig. 14-2.

area frequently result in paralysis of all four extremities (quadriplegia).

There are a number of congenital abnormalities that can affect the region of the craniovertebral or cervicomedullary junction. These include the three types of Chiari malformations, basilar invagination, achondroplasia, Morquio syndrome, Down syndrome, and Klippel-Feil syndrome. The primarily deleterious effect that each of these congenital abnormalities has on the CNS is to narrow the space normally occupied by the medulla and upper cervical spinal cord. This area of the CNS is so vitally important that an abnormality in this region is frequently considered a medical emergency. However, it is also a part of the MR scan that is exceedingly easy to inadvertently overlook. This is because it is at the top of the cervical spine study, and frequently is not thought of as being part of the cervical spine examination, while at the same time being at the bottom of the cranial MRI. The MR technologist can be very effective in evaluating this region, since it is commonly from a midline sagittal view of either the brain or the cervical spine that additional images are programmed. Attention to the appearance of the foramen magnum and upper cervical spinal

canal combined with a working knowledge of "normal" is all that is required. Figure 14-8A and B demonstrates the normal (A) and the abnormal (B) appearance of the craniocervical (cervicomedullary) junction in a patient with a malformation that narrows the normal size of the foramen magnum and upper cervical spinal canal.

Infections and neoplasms can also result in compression of vital brainstem or upper cervical spinal structures. In these types of disease processes, the abnormality may arise from adjacent tissues and compress a region of the CNS, or it may arise from within the brainstem or spinal cord. Because the space is small and confined by hard bone, the result is often the same. That is, there is insufficient room within the confines of the foramen magnum or spinal canal (see Fig. 14-9).

The postoperative spinal MRI is among the most difficult of examinations, and unlike the situation with the

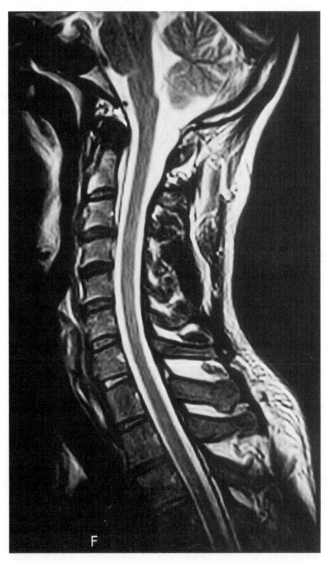

Figure 14-2   Sagittal SE T2-weighted MR (TR 3000, TE 96) demonstrating the normal appearance of the cervical spine. Note that the spinal cord is seen as a relatively lower signal against the brighter surrounding CSF. Compare to Fig. 14-1.

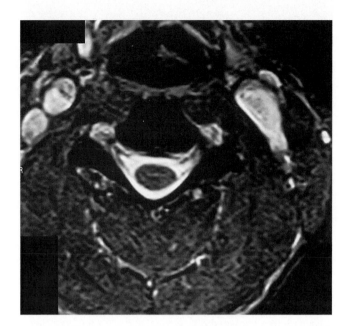

Figure 14-3   Axial GRE T2-weighted MR (TR 877, TE 16, FA 35) demonstrating the normal appearance of the cervical spine. Note that the spinal cord and nerve roots are seen as a relatively lower signal against the brighter surrounding CSF.

lumbar spine, MRI contrast agents do not appear to add significantly to diagnostic efficacy. The study is frequently performed in an unhappy and perhaps uncooperative patient who suffers from continued pain. In addition, there may be artifacts from metallic implants, wire sutures, and even remaining metal fragments from the bone drills that are used during surgery (see Fig. 14-10). These small or even microscopic particles of metal can leave significant distortion artifacts on the MRI examination. When just the slightest motion is added, the technologist may become very frustrated in the attempt to obtain a good-quality study. Working at a slightly slower pace and reassuring the patient may be of benefit. However, even the most valiant attempts to obtain a truly good-quality postoperative cervical spine MRI may fail. Adding contrast rarely improves the quality of the examination, and in some patients a marginal examination may be all that is possible. Unfortunately, this often results in complaints from the physician who must interpret the study as well as from the referring clinicians. Although there may be an added time requirement for scanning, one method of improving some of these postoperative cervical spine studies is to avoid gradient recalled (GRE) sequences, which have increased sensitivity to both motion and metal (see Fig. 14-11A–C).

The evaluation of spinal tumors will almost certainly involve MRI as one of the primary examinations, and in many instances this will be the initial method of diagnosis. The neoplasm may arise from directly within the spinal cord or from the tissues surrounding the spinal cord. When the disease process begins outside of the spinal cord, consideration must be given to the extent of any compression of the spinal cord. Direct compression of the spinal cord, especially in the cervical region, is usually considered a

medical emergency. Depending on the nature of the compression, immediate surgical intervention is often required. The most common neoplasm arising outside of the spinal cord but resulting in compression of the spinal cord is a metastatic lesion. Typically, the metastasis will begin in the adjacent vertebral body and subsequently grow until it compresses the spinal canal and spinal cord. It is important to remember that a positive MRI for spinal metastatic disease in one part of the spine, such as the cervical region, makes the likelihood of additional involvement of other levels, such as the thoracic and lumbar spine, much higher. Therefore, some centers routinely perform screening sagittal T1 MRI scans of the entire spine in these patients, since this exam is both the most rapid and the most diagnostic for spinal metastases (see Fig. 14-12).

Additional neoplasms that may affect the spinal cord and spinal canal include ependymomas and astrocytomas,

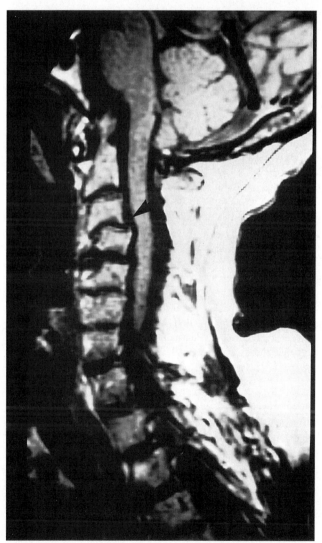

Figure 14-4   Sagittal SE T1-weighted MR (TR 600, TE 20) demonstrating the appearance of advanced degenerative changes of the cervical spine. Note that the spinal cord is seen as a relatively higher signal against the darker surrounding CSF and that there is subluxation of C3 on C4 (anterior displacement). Compare to Fig. 14-1.

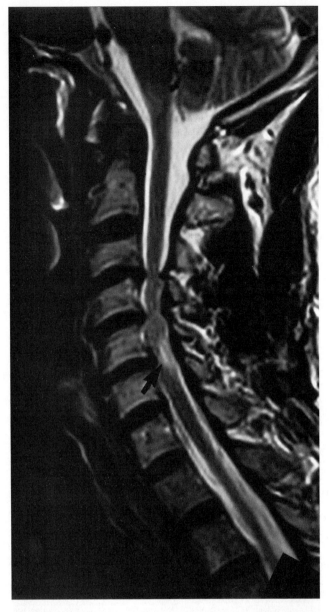

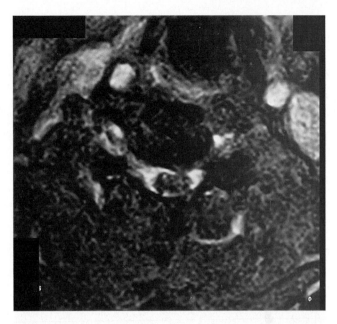

Figure 14-6 Axial GRE T2-weighted MR (TR 877, TE 16, FA 35) demonstrating the narrowing of the left neural foramen secondary to a herniated disc (*arrow*) and associated degenerative disease. Compare to Fig. 14-6.

Figure 14-5 Sagittal SE T2-weighted MR (TR 3000, TE 96) demonstrating marked narrowing of the cervical spinal canal with spinal cord compression. Note that the spinal cord is seen as a relatively lower signal against the brighter surrounding CSF and that there is a focus of high signal within the spinal cord from ischemia secondary to pressure (*arrow*).

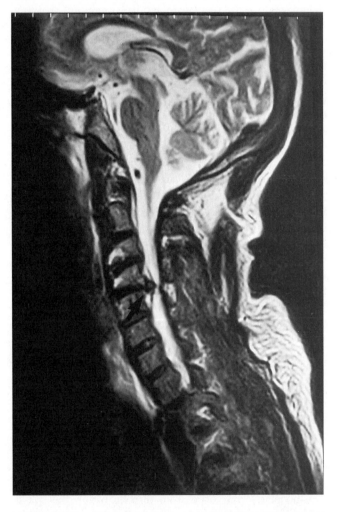

Figure 14-7 Sagittal SE T2-weighted MR (TR 3000, TE 96) demonstrating marked narrowing of the cervical spinal canal secondary to a herniated disc (*arrow*). Note that the herniated disc is seen as a relatively lower signal against the brighter surrounding CSF.

162

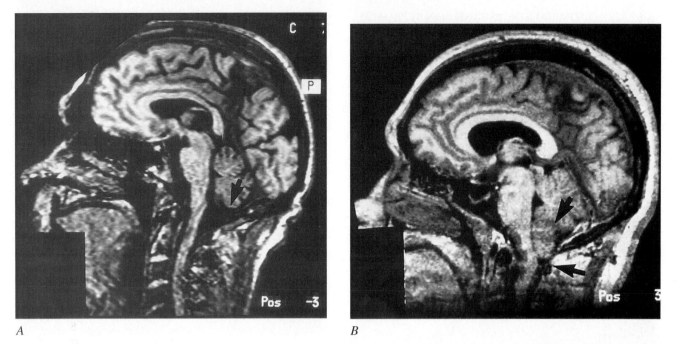

A

B

Figure 14-8 *A.* Sagittal GRE T1-weighted MR (TR 40, TE 6, FA 40) demonstrating the normal appearance of the foramen magnum (*arrow*) with dark CSF surrounding the brainstem and upper spinal cord. Compare to Fig. 14-8. *B.* Sagittal GRE T1-weighted MR (TR 10, TE 4, FA 10) demonstrating an abnormality at the level of the foramen magnum (*lower arrow*) with the brainstem deviated (kinked) anteriorly and compression of this space by low-lying cerebellar tonsils (*upper arrow*). Compare to Fig. 14-7.

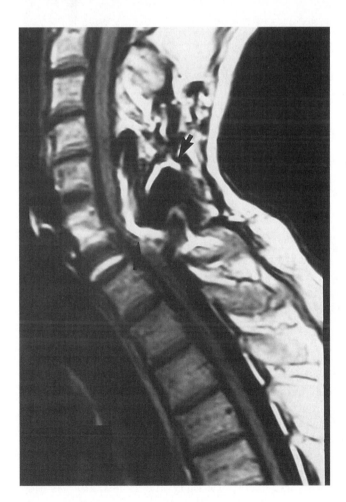

Figure 14-10 Sagittal SE T1-weighted MR (TR 500, TE 16) demonstrating apparent narrowing of cervical spinal canal. Note the metallic artifact (*arrow*) and the extensive postoperative changes. Compare to Fig. 14-11.

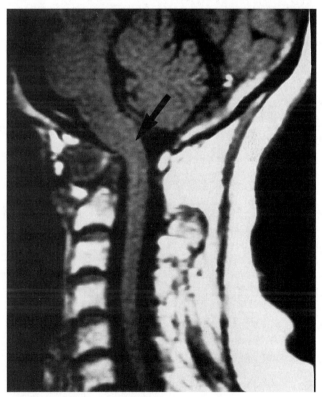

Figure 14-9 Sagittal SE T1-weighted MR (TR 600, TE 11) demonstrating severe narrowing of the foramen magnum and upper cervical spinal canal from a large soft tissue mass (*white arrow*). This disease process is secondary to advanced inflammatory change (pannus) associated with rheumatoid arthritis. Note that the spinal cord is seen as a relatively higher signal against the darker surrounding CSF and that the upper spinal cord is kinked at this level (*black arrow*).

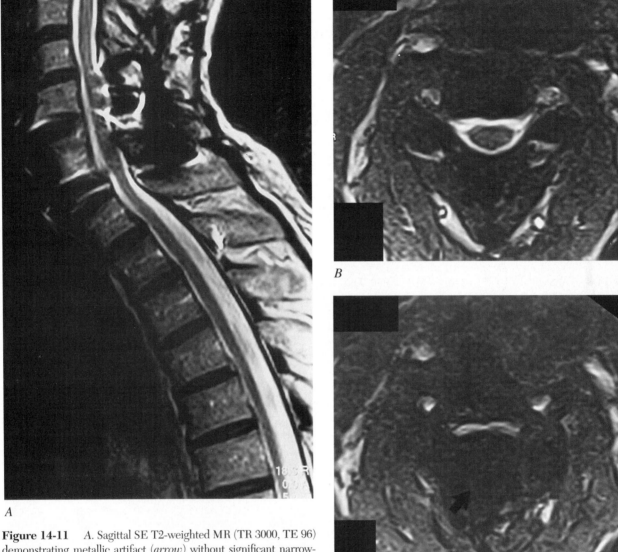

A

B

C

Figure 14-11 *A*. Sagittal SE T2-weighted MR (TR 3000, TE 96) demonstrating metallic artifact (*arrow*) without significant narrowing of the cervical spinal canal. Compare to Figs. 14-10 and 14-11*B* and *C*. Note that there is very little distortion in spite of the metallic artifact when SE sequences are used. *B*. Axial GRE T2-weighted MR (TR 1367, TE 16, FA 35) demonstrating the normal appearance of the cervical spinal canal. Note that the spinal cord and nerve roots are seen as a relatively lower signal against the brighter surrounding CSF. Compare to Fig. 14-11*A* and *C*. *C*. Axial GRE T2-weighted MR (TR 1367, TE 16, FA 35) demonstrating complete loss of the normal appearance of the cervical spinal canal due to metallic artifact (*arrow*). Compare to Fig. 14-11*A* and *B*.

which commonly arise from within the spinal cord (see Fig. 14-13). Tumors such as meningiomas, neurofibromas, and schwannomas will more commonly compress the spinal cord as a result of narrowing of the spinal canal. However, degenerative disease and disc herniations are much more common causes of spinal canal narrowing or spinal cord compression than spinal neoplasms (see Fig. 14-5).

Infections of the spinal cord or nerve roots are also more likely to begin in the adjacent structures. Osteomyelitis of the vertebral bodies, disc space infections (discitis), and paraspinous soft tissue abscesses are most often the cause of infections that compress or directly involve the spinal cord and nerve roots. Osteomyelitis of the

spinal vertebral bodies is usually due to the spread of infection from some other part of the body, such as the skin, genitourinary tract, or lungs. This spread is frequently through the bloodstream, and therefore can arise from any other part of the body. More localized infections, such as a retropharyngeal or paraspinous abscess, can invade the spinal canal directly. All of these infections are considered extremely serious, and when the infection moves directly into the spinal canal, the results may be catastrophic. Not only can the spinal cord or nerve roots be compressed, but if the infection enters the subdural or subarachnoid space, it can rapidly spread to any part of the central nervous system. This type of spread will fre-

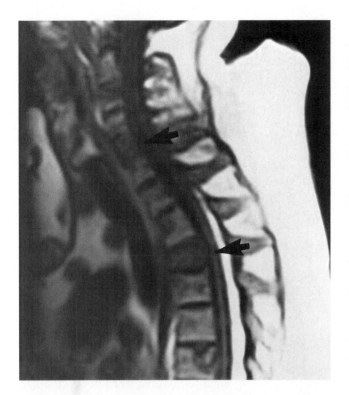

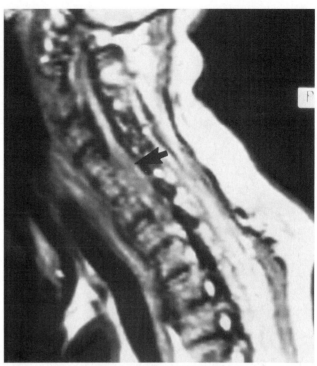

Figure 14-12 Sagittal SE T1-weighted MR (TR 438, TE 20) demonstrating low signal from vertebral body metastatic disease at C5 (*upper arrow*) and low signal as well as narrowing of spinal canal at T2 (*lower arrow*) from metastatic disease that has spread from the vertebral body into the spinal canal. Findings of spinal metastatic disease in one part of the spine are often associated with metastatic disease at other levels.

Figure 14-13 Sagittal SE proton-density-weighted MR (TR 2010, TE 22) demonstrating abnormal expansion of the cervical spinal cord (*arrow*) from a spinal cord tumor. Note how this compares to a lesion compressing the spinal cord as illustrated in Fig. 14-12.

quently result in severe neurologic impairment or even death.

Although less common, vascular abnormalities can lead to clinical symptoms referable to the cervical spine. Aneurysms, arteriovenous malformations, and even spinal cord infarctions do occur in the cervical region as well as in all parts of the spine. In addition to bleeding, aneurysms and arteriovenous malformations can cause direct pressure on the spinal cord, due again to the small, confined space of the spinal canal. When bleeding occurs, it can result in compression of the spinal cord by a hematoma, direct hemorrhage into the spinal cord, or irritation of the blood vessels supplying the spinal cord. This irritation can lead to spasm of the blood vessels and is one cause of spinal cord infarction. Additional causes of spinal cord infarction include atherosclerotic disease, compression of blood vessels by infectious or neoplastic processes, and trauma. In general, spinal cord infarctions are rare, especially when compared to the frequency of cerebral infarctions. This is because the blood supply to the spinal cord is quite generous and redundant. Nonetheless, spinal cord infarctions do occur, and MRI is the most sensitive method available to confirm the diagnosis.

MRI of the cervical spine is particularly effective in the evaluation of trauma, and is currently the only imaging method for directly visualizing the extent of soft tissue injury to the spine. This is very important, since soft tissue injury and not fractures accounts for most of the danger to vital functions that accompanies spinal trauma. A loss of the stability provided by the ligaments, tendons, and muscles that support the spine most frequently leads to direct injury of the spinal cord and nerve roots. Therefore, MR is rapidly becoming the diagnostic procedure of choice for the evaluation of the injured spine. In some institutions, all patients with significant cervical spine injuries undergo an urgent MRI study to determine the extent of injury to supporting tissues and the spinal cord. The primary limitation of MRI in the evaluation of spine trauma is in the assessment of bone injuries. An additional problem may be the metallic devices that are often needed to provide adequate life support for severely injured patients. This includes endotracheal tubes, traction devices, and some types of ventilators. It is also important to know that most "wood" spine boards are reinforced with metal bars, and a Plexiglas spine board may be required if the patient is to remain immobilized on a spine board during the MRI examination.

Although any part of the spinal column may be evaluated with MRI following trauma, the most common area to be examined is the cervical spine. This is because of both the frequency of cervical spine injuries and the need for accurate assessment of the cervical spine before the patient can be safely immobilized. MRI is superior to both plain films and CT for the evaluation of soft tissue injuries of the

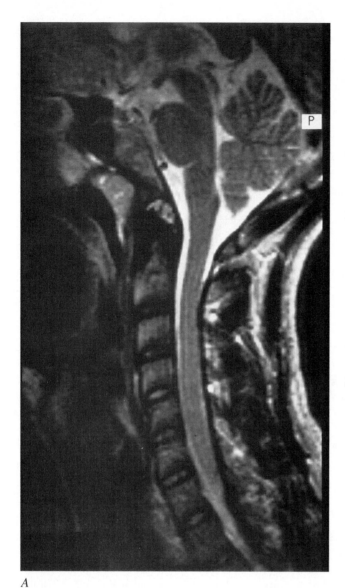

A

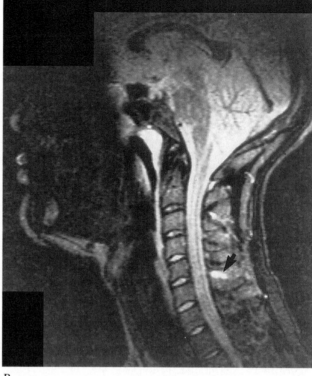

B

Figure 14-14 *A.* Sagittal SE T2-weighted MR (TR 3500, TE 103) demonstrating no definite abnormality of the cervical spine. *B.* Sagittal STIR MR (TR 1800, TE 20, IR 180) demonstrating abnormal interspinous ligamentous signal in this patient with a neck injury from a motor vehicle accident.

spine, and can be used as a means to "guide" the CT examination following trauma. Areas that demonstrate abnormal signal intensity on MRI are more likely to show fractures on subsequent CT studies, especially when thin-section CT is performed through the levels that are abnormal on MRI. The abnormal signal intensity identified on MRI following spinal trauma is best visualized on short-TI inversion recovery (STIR) sequences. The STIR examination provides excellent tissue contrast while the normal fat signal is suppressed, so that abnormalities show up as bright signal against a dark background. These lesions will rarely, if ever, be noted on standard T1 sequences, and are also easily overlooked on standard T2 studies. In fact, without the use of STIR, severe ligamentous injury can be easily overlooked on the MRI following spinal trauma (see Fig. 14-14*A* and *B*).

MRI of the cervical spine is an extremely valuable tool in the assessment of a broad range of degenerative, neurologic, bony, and posttraumatic disorders. Because of the prevalence of degenerative spine disease, the cervical spinal MRI may be one of the most common examinations performed in any active MRI center. A working

knowledge of the anatomy and pathology of the cervical spine should enhance both the quality and the effectiveness of this examination. The MRI technologist can further the positive impact of these studies by being alert to pathologic changes that may require the use of additional pulse sequences or a contrast agent.

Suggested Readings

Orrison WW Jr: *Introduction to Neuroimaging.* Boston, Little Brown, 1989.

Modic MT, Masaryk TJ, Ross JS (eds.): *Magnetic Resonance Imaging of the Spine,* 2nd ed. St. Louis, MO, Mosby, 1994.

Latchaw RE (ed.): *MR and CT Imaging of the Head, Neck, and Spine,* vols. 1 and 2. St. Louis, MO, Mosby, 1991.

Ramsey RG: *Neuroradiology,* 3rd ed. Philadelphia, PA, Saunders, 1994.

15

Thoracic
Spine Imaging

The evaluation of the thoracic spine is similar in many regards to that of the cervical spine. However, the thoracic spine is more uniform in the size and shape of the vertebral bodies, and is the part of the spinal canal in which there is a contiguous segment of the spinal cord (see Fig. 15-1A and B). The disease processes that affect the thoracic spine are identical to those that affect the cervical spine; however, the frequency of involvement is different. For example, the most common reason for performing a cervical or lumbar spine MRI is typically to evaluate degenerative disease, whereas the thoracic spine MRI is more likely to be an evaluation of possible metastatic disease, infection, or an abnormality of the spinal cord.

One disease condition that may often involve the thoracic spinal cord is syringomyelia or syringohydromyelia. Hydromyelia is enlargement of the central canal of the spinal cord, whereas syringomyelia is cavitation of the spinal cord separate from the central canal. These two conditions may coexist, and it is usually not possible to differentiate between them on imaging studies. Therefore, some authors prefer the term *syringohydromyelia* to describe a condition in which there is abnormal CSF signal identified within the substance of the spinal cord. More often than not, the technologist will encounter a request that simply states, "rule out syrinx" or "rule out syringomyelia." In this instance, the referring clinician is looking for the condition of syringohydromyelia. This problem is often related to trauma, but frequently the clinical symptoms will not begin until several years after the traumatic event. Other causes of syringohydromyelia include tumors, spinal cord infarction, and congenital anomalies.

The symptoms that patients with syringohydromyelia exhibit can be quite varied, and include severe pain, weakness, muscle atrophy, skin abnormalities, joint abnormalities, and unusual sensory changes. It is often these sensory changes that lead the clinician to suspect a diagnosis of syringohydromyelia. The sensory loss is described clinically as "dissociated," so that, for example, there may be loss of sensations of pain and temperature with preservation of the sense of touch. The symptoms may be unilateral or bilateral, and may change dramatically over short periods of time.

MRI examination of the spinal cord is the diagnostic procedure of choice for syringohydromyelia, and the diagnosis is often obvious on the sagittal T1- or T2-weighted sequences (see Fig. 15-2). However, it is also important to obtain axial images through the levels of abnormality or suspected abnormality, since eccentric areas of syringohydromyelia may be difficult to visualize on sagittal images and may also be obscured by partial volume with the adjacent CSF within the surrounding spinal canal (see Fig. 15-3). When an area of syringohydromyelia is identified in one area of the spinal cord, it is common practice to evaluate the entire spinal cord, since "skip areas" are frequently encountered. Since syringohydromyelia may involve any region from the brainstem to the tip of the spinal cord, imaging of the posterior fossa of the cranium is also included. In addition, a contrast-enhanced study to exclude an associated neoplasm is indicated in most cases. This can become a long and involved scan, especially when multiple levels of the spinal cord must be evaluated with axial images. It is important for the technologist to keep in mind that treatment for the patient often depends on the exact location and full extent of the regions of syringohydromyelia. Therefore, a complete and careful study is indicated, even if it is difficult and time consuming.

167

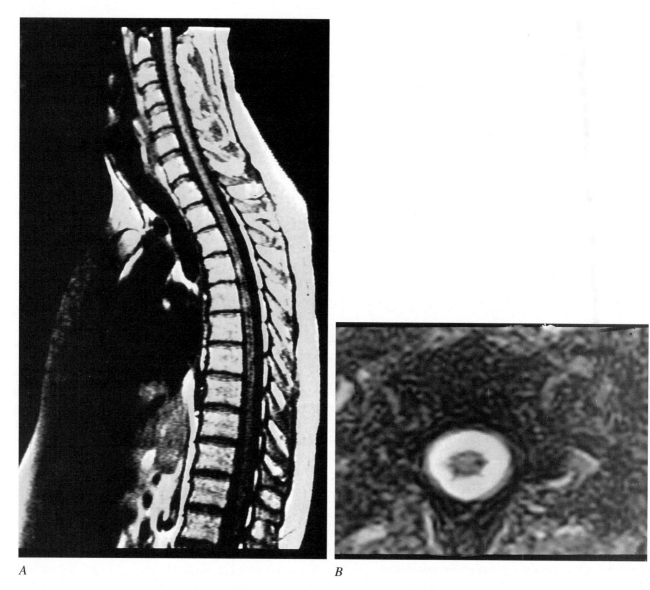

A

B

Figure 15-1   *A.* Sagittal SE T1-weighted MR (TR 450, TE 15) demonstrating the normal appearance of the cervical and thoracic spine. Note that the spinal cord is seen as a relatively higher signal against the darker surrounding CSF. *B.* Axial GRE T2-weighted MR (TR 1367, TE 16, FA 35) demonstrating the normal appearance of the thoracic spine. Note that the spinal cord and nerve roots are seen as a relatively lower signal against the brighter surrounding CSF.

Spinal metastatic disease is quite common, and occurs in about 10 percent of patients with cancer. Spinal metastatic disease can affect any level of the spine and any part of the spine. However, metastatic cancer that has spread to the epidural spinal canal often results in neurologic symptoms, which lead to the need for an MRI examination. This type of cancer spread is more often located in the thoracic spine, with approximately 70 percent occurring here. About 15 percent is found in the cervical spine, and another 15 percent in the lumbar. Therefore, the MR technologist is likely to be in a position to evaluate patients for metastases to the thoracic spine on a regular basis.

The types of cancer that most commonly lead to spinal metastases include lung, breast, prostate, uterine, lymphoma, and myeloma. Regardless of the type of cancer that has spread to the spine or the level within the spine, there are generally similar changes that are identified on MRI. This means that MRI can often detect the changes that represent metastatic disease to the spine, but is seldom effective in determining exactly what kind of cancer caused the abnormality. This is usually referred to as high sensitivity (finding the abnormality), but with low specificity (determining the type of cancer). The typical findings on MRI are involvement of the spinal vertebrae with or without associated abnormalities of the adjacent soft tissues.

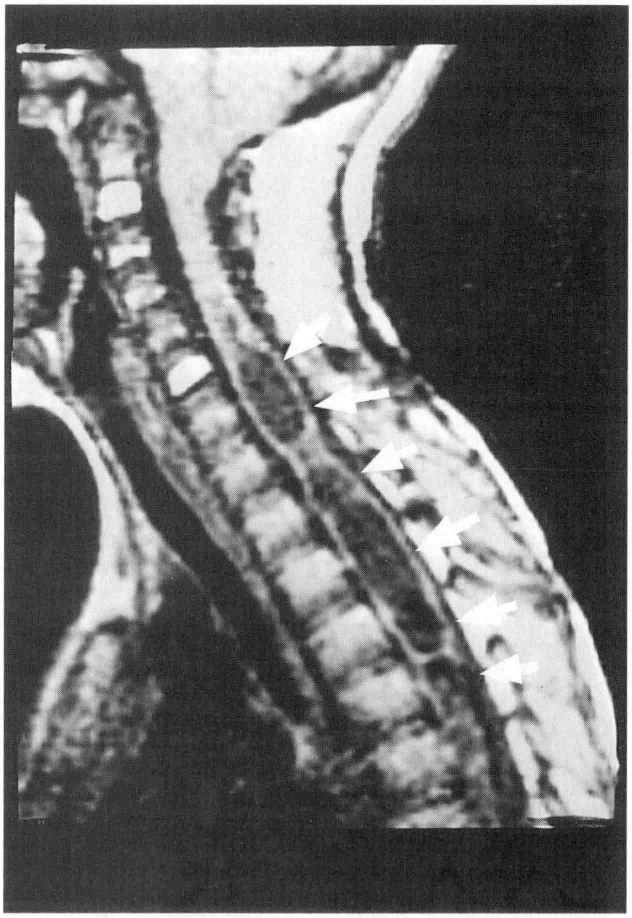

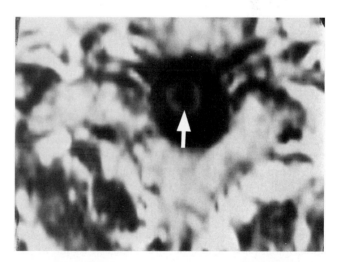

ment of this patient. Care in filming and calling this condition to the attention of the staff physician may be the only way in which this problem can be recognized (see Fig. 15-5). Note that the signal intensity of all of the vertebral bodies in total metastatic involvement of the spine is uniform but of *lower signal* than that of the intervertebral discs. Normally, the intervertebral disc signal is lower than that of the vertebral bodies because of the presence of fat within the marrow space. However, this fat is replaced by metastatic disease, with the result being a decrease in signal intensity to a level lower than that of the intervertebral disc. Therefore, *whenever the MR technologist identifies a T1-weighted scan of the spine in which the vertebral body signal is uniformly lower than that of the intervertebral discs, this condition should be brought to the attention of the attending physician.* In addition, the filming of this case must be done in the same manner as for the normal spine in order to avoid decreasing the appearance of the metastatic disease. Changing the window and level in order to make the spine "look right" can make this condition much more difficult to recognize.

The appearance of metastatic disease on T2-weighted sequences is quite variable, and the result may even be no significant signal change within the vertebral bodies. Unlike for the brain and other organ systems, where T2-weighted sequences may be the most diagnostic, in the evaluation of metastatic disease to the vertebral column, T2 sequences are notoriously unreliable (see Fig. 15-6). Likewise, gadolinium can be problematic in the evaluation of metastatic disease to the vertebral bodies. The enhancement of the tumor tissue will often bring the signal up to match that of the normal fat within the bone marrow, and "mask" the findings on T1 sequences (see Fig.

Figure 15-2 Sagittal SE T1-weighted MR (TR 600, TE 20) demonstrating the appearance of a large and multilevel syrinx of the lower cervical and upper thoracic spinal cord (*arrows*). The spinal cord is seen as a relatively higher signal against the darker surrounding CSF, and there is also a darker central area within the spinal cord representing the syrinx. (Compare to Fig. 15-3.) Note that the "white" vertebral bodies are secondary to radiation change with fatty replacement of the bone marrow at these levels.

The MRI sequence that is generally of most value in the initial evaluation of the spine for metastatic disease is the T1-weighted sagittal examination. On this study, the diseased segments of the vertebral column will appear as areas of relative signal loss. That is, the regions of metastatic involvement will be dark compared to the rest of the vertebral bodies and intervertebral discs (see Fig. 15-4). *There is a very important exception to this appearance, of which the MR technologist should beware!* In patients with total involvement of the spinal vertebral bodies by metastatic disease, the signal within the vertebral bodies will be uniform. This means that relative to other vertebral bodies, there will be no difference in signal. *This condition is very easily overlooked by anyone reviewing the scan.* Therefore, the opportunity exists for the MR technologist to make a very real difference in the manage-

Figure 15-3 Axial SE T1-weighted MR (TR 800, TE 15) demonstrating the appearance of a syrinx involving the thoracic spinal cord (*arrow*). The spinal cord is seen as a relatively higher signal against the darker surrounding CSF, and there is also a darker central area (*arrow*) within the spinal cord representing the syrinx. (Compare to Fig. 15-2.)

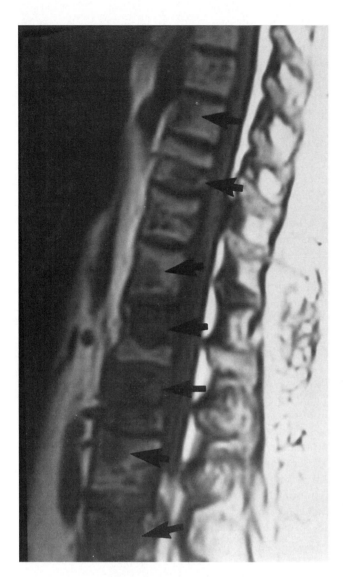

Figure 15-4 Sagittal SE T1-weighted MR (TR 438, TE 20) demonstrating the appearance of metastases involving the thoracic and lumbar spine at multiple levels (*arrows*).

15-7*A* and *B*). Therefore, performing gadolinium-only scans for the evaluation of the spine is fraught with difficulties. However, gadolinium is extremely effective in the evaluation of metastatic disease to the epidural space, soft tissues, and spinal cord (see Fig. 15-8*A* and *B*).

In order to decrease the need for gadolinium in the evaluation of spinal metastatic disease, the use of short-TI inversion recovery (STIR) sequences has been added to the routine spine survey by some centers. The STIR sequence provides not only increased signal in the epidural spinal metastatic lesions, but also increased signal in the soft tissues and the vertebral column (see Fig. 15-9). The advantages of STIR include increased tissue contrast, particularly for neoplastic and inflammatory conditions, and a decrease in the need for gadolinium. The primary disadvantage is relatively low resolution and motion sensitivity. For this reason, the STIR sequence has been referred to

as the "nuclear medicine scan of MR" because of its high contrast and relatively low resolution compared to other MR studies. However, when compared to nuclear medicine examinations, the resolution remains significantly better.

It is important for everyone involved in the evaluation of possible spinal disease to remember that the patient is often in significant pain. The level of the patient's discomfort can be quite exaggerated by movement and the positions required during the MRI study. Unfortunately, even with the most modern MRI scanners, the manner in which the patient must be placed within the magnetic field remains limited, the length of the scan is at least 15 to 30 min or longer, and the patient must be transferred to and from the scan table. This can be a miserable ordeal for both the patient and the technologist, but keeping in mind how terribly painful this

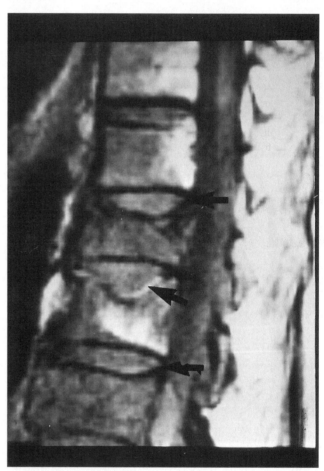

Figure 15-5 Sagittal SE T1-weighted MR (TR 438, TE 20) demonstrating the appearance of metastases involving the thoracic and lumbar spine at multiple levels. Note that the vertebral bodies are diffusely low in signal and that the intervertebral discs are of higher signal than the adjacent vertebral bodies (*arrows*). This is indicative of diffuse metastatic disease, and the only clue may be the alteration in higher signal of the discs relative to the vertebral bodies on T1 scans. (Compare to Fig. 15-6.)

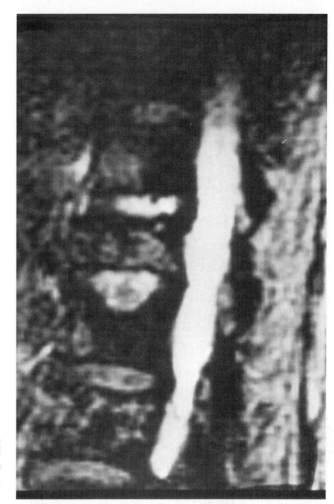

Figure 15-6 Sagittal GRE T2-weighted MR (TR 800, TE 35, FA 10) demonstrating increased signal in parts of the vertebral bodies but a relatively normal appearance of other areas of the thoracic spine in a patient with diffuse vertebral body metastases. (Compare to Fig. 15-5.)

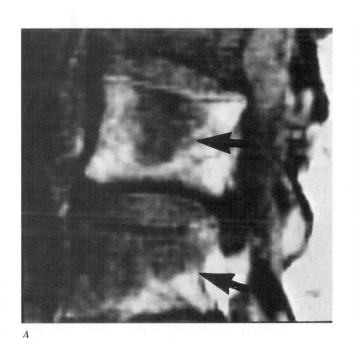

A

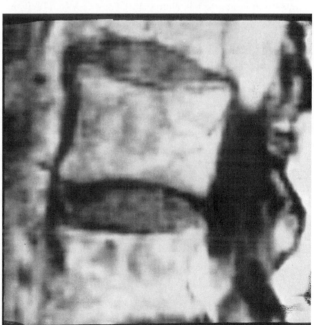

B

Figure 15-7 *A.* Sagittal SE T1-weighted MR (TR 800, TE 20) demonstrating the appearance of metastases involving the thoracic and lumbar spine *(arrows)*. *B.* Sagittal SE gadolinium-enhanced T1-weighted MR (TR 800, TE 20) demonstrating loss of the appearance of the metastases involving the thoracic and lumbar spine *(arrows)*. Note how "normal" the vertebral bodies appear on this scan compared to the pre-gadolinium scan in *A.*

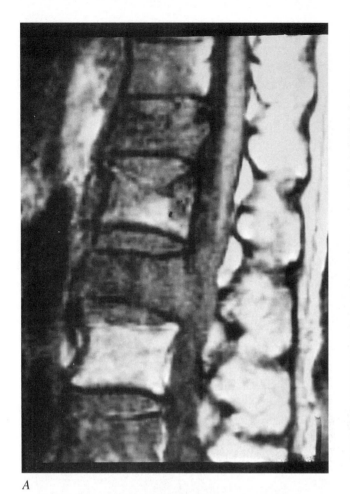

A

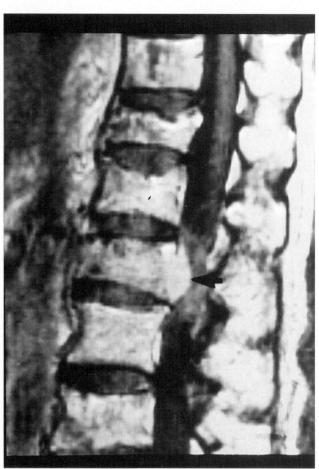

B

Figure 15-8 *A.* Sagittal SE T1-weighted MR (TR 800, TE 20) demonstrating the appearance of multiple metastases involving the thoracic and lumbar spine. Note that the one vertebral body of higher signal is the only "normal" vertebral body on this image. (Compare to *B.*) *B.* Sagittal SE gadolinium-enhanced T1-weighted MR (TR 800, TE 20) demonstrating loss of the appearance of the metastases involving the thoracic and lumbar spinal vertebral bodies. Note how "normal" the vertebral bodies appear on this scan compared to the pre-gadolinium scan in *A.* However, also note how much more obvious the epidural extension of the metastatic process becomes *(arrow)* when the lesion is enhanced with gadolinium.

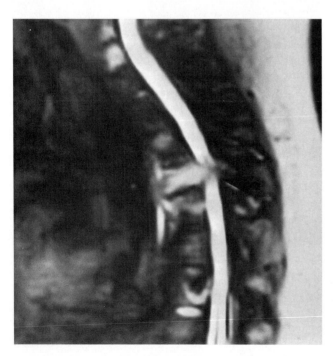

Figure 15-9 Sagittal STIR MR (TR 4646, TE 32, TI 150) demonstrating narrowing of the spinal canal from metastatic disease *(arrow)*. Also note the involvement of other levels of the spine as depicted by the abnormal increased signal. On STIR sequences the areas of abnormality are bright as compared to the decreased signal seen on T1 sequences. (Compare to Figs. 15-4, 15-5, 15-7A, and 15-8A.)

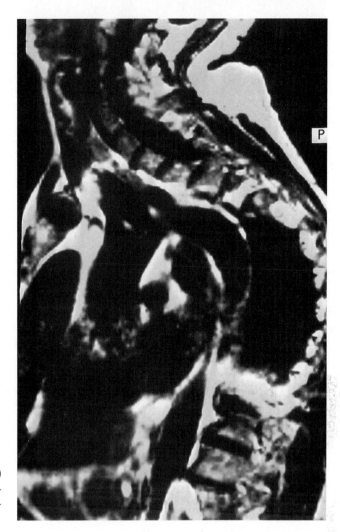

Figure 15-10 Sagittal SE T1-weighted MR (TR 350, TE 15) demonstrating marked curvature of the spine of this severely debilitated patient. This is the type of patient who may be particularly challenging for the MR technologist.

process can be for the patient should enable the technologist to be more compassionate. When the disease process results in spinal cord compression, the most frequent patient problems, in addition to pain, are weakness and autonomic dysfunction. This results in the MR technologist's nightmare: the often elderly, frail, tender, paralyzed, and incontinent patient! However, this is the same patient who requires the best of the MR technologist in every regard. The speed and quality of the MR examination in this instance may determine whether this patient will ever walk again or recover control of bowel and bladder functions. These studies may not be the MR technologist's favorite, but they are among the most important scans that the technologist will ever perform (see Fig. 15-10).

Suggested Reading

Orrison WW Jr: *Introduction to Neuroimaging.* Boston, Little Brown, 1989.

16

Lumbar Spine Imaging

The MRI examination of the lumbar spine may be the single most common study performed in many imaging centers. The lumbar spine MRI is most often performed for the evaluation of possible degenerative changes or to exclude lumbar disc disease. The examination is frequently performed in patients who are experiencing severe pain, and patient tolerance is often a factor in the quality of the MRI obtained. Anything that the technologist can do to improve patient comfort during the exam will probably enhance the quality of the MRI. However, making the patient comfortable may also mean positioning the patient in a manner that will decrease the amount of pathology visualized. From a practical standpoint, making the patient comfortable usually outweighs the possibility that such manipulation of the spine will obviate pathology. In general, simply placing a pillow or other form of bolster under the patient's knees will suffice to allow for completion of the MRI study.

The image that is most often of primary benefit in the evaluation of the lumbar spine is the sagittal T2- or T2°-weighted sequence. The T1-weighted exam is also important to obtain, since, as was demonstrated in the discussion of the thoracic spine (see Chap. 15), this may be the only sequence that will show evidence of metastatic disease. These sequences will demonstrate the relationship of the vertebral bodies and intervertebral disc spaces to the remainder of the spinal canal, and to each other. In addition, this exam will typically show the inferior aspect of the spinal cord and the cauda equina. The amount of hydration of the intervertebral disc and the overall size of the spinal canal can readily be assessed on these images (see Fig. 16-1A and B.)

Axial images are also obtained, and these will show the vertebral body or intervertebral disc anteriorly, the CSF-filled spinal canal, the nerve roots within the spinal canal, and the adjacent soft tissues (see Fig. 16-2). Axial images may be obtained as a block of straight sequential images or angled to the disc space (see Fig. 16-3). When the images are aligned parallel to the disc space, it is important for the technologist to be certain that true parallel scans are obtained (see Fig. 16-4). The advantages of scanning parallel to the disc space include the ability to visualize all intervertebral discs on a single acquisition and less partial volume effect from the adjacent vertebral bodies. Axial images may be obtained with T1 or T2 sequences. The T1 sequences generally will not show the spinal canal and nerve roots as well as the T2 or T2° sequences (see Fig. 16-2).

Narrowing of the spinal canal is frequently referred to as *spinal stenosis*. This condition can result from extension of the intervertebral disc (disc bulge or herniation), bony overgrowth of the vertebral body (osteocyte formation), hypertrophy of the facet joints, ligament hypertrophy (ligamentum flavum enlargement), excessive fat within the spinal canal (epidural lipomatosis), and/or congenital narrowing of the spinal canal (short pedicle stenosis). Any or all of these conditions may contribute to spinal stenosis in a given patient (see Fig. 16-5A and B). Spinal stenosis is often evaluated as being mild, moderate, or severe.

Mild spinal stenosis is quite common, and the back pain that may be associated is frequently due to the accompanying conditions, such as osteophyte formation or facet hypertrophy. Moderate and severe spinal stenosis represent much more serious clinical conditions that may be debilitating for the patient. Lumbar spinal stenosis is associated with a clinical condition referred to as *neurogenic claudication*. The pain is often bilateral, radicular in nature (follows nerve roots), and accompanied by sensory and motor deficits (loss of sensation and weakness). The

175

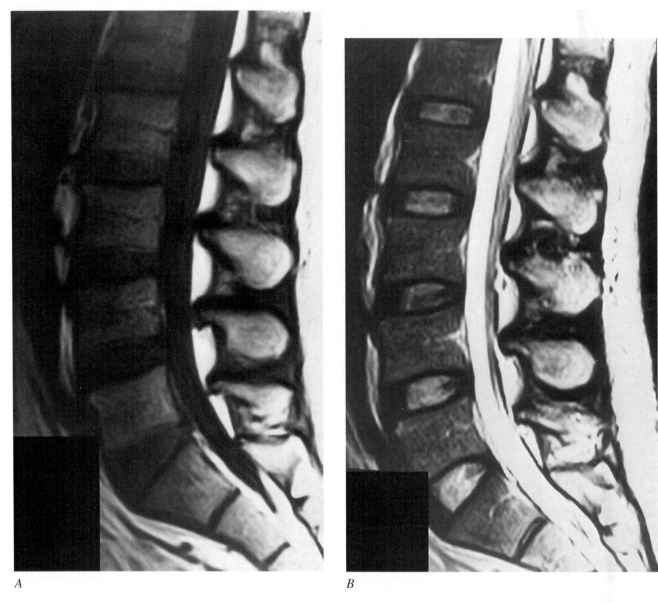

A   *B*

Figure 16-1   *A*. Sagittal SE T1-weighted MR (TR 500, TE 20) demonstrating the normal appearance of the lumbar spine. Note that the spinal canal is seen as a relatively lower signal containing the darker CSF and that the intervertebral discs are also dark (compare to *B*). *B*. Sagittal SE T2-weighted MR (TR 4600, TE 112) demonstrating the normal appearance of the lumbar spine. Note that the spinal canal is seen as a relatively higher signal containing the brighter CSF and that the intervertebral discs are also bright (compare to *A*).

patient may report that the condition is actually made worse by standing and/or walking, but relieved by lying down. These patients may seem to the MR technologist as if they are malingering, since they will be in severe pain while waiting for the examination, but immediately improve when lying down for the scan. They may actually appear to be "cured" by the scan, when in reality their pain will return shortly after they leave the scan area.

When one vertebral body is displaced anteriorly over the vertebral body below, the condition is referred to as *spondylolisthesis*. Degenerative spondylolisthesis is usually related to degenerative changes in the facet joints.

Degenerative disc disease also contributes to this condition, which is made more severe by the narrowing of the intervertebral disc space that accompanies degenerative disc disease. Spondylolisthesis is commonly "graded" based on the degree of vertebral body displacement. The sagittal MRI of the spine will show the amount that the vertebral body is shifted. When less than one-fourth of the vertebral body is displaced, the grade is I. Displacement of the vertebral body to the midway point is graded as II, and three-fourths displacement is referred to as grade III. A grade IV displacement represents complete dislocation of the upper vertebral body over the lower

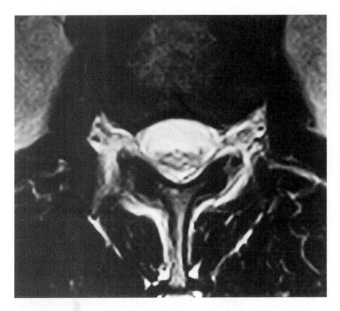

Figure 16-2 Axial SE T2-weighted MR (TR 4857, TE 112) demonstrating the normal appearance of the lumbar spine. Note that the spinal canal is seen as a relatively higher signal containing the brighter CSF and that the intervertebral discs are also bright.

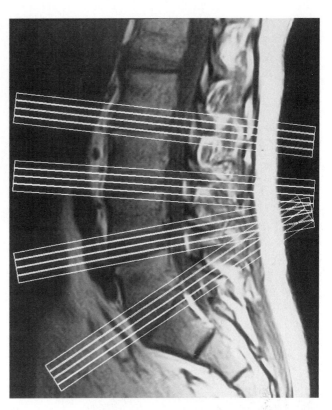

Figure 16-4 Sagittal SE T1-weighted MR (TR 500, TE 20) demonstrating the sections obtained when axial scans are obtained parallel to the intervertebral disc space.

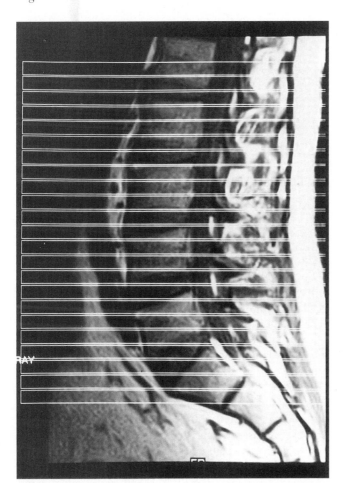

Figure 16-3 Sagittal SE T1-weighted MR (TR 500, TE 20) demonstrating the sections obtained when axial scans are obtained in a "stacked" manner.

(see Fig. 16-6). When the vertebral body above is positioned posteriorly on the vertebral body below, the term *retrolesthesis* is used to describe this change (Fig. 16-7).

When there is degeneration of the intervertebral disc, there are corresponding signal changes on the MRI. These signal changes are in part due to the loss of hydration within the intervertebral disc. As a result, the disc degeneration visualized on MRI is usually a combination of decreased intervertebral disc space height and decreased intervertebral disc signal (see Fig. 16-8). This signal loss is due in part to dehydration of the disc itself, and may also be a reflection of changes in the manner in which water is held within the disc space.

The classification of degenerative changes within the spine has been the subject of great controversy. This is particularly the case when the intervertebral disc extends beyond the normal confines of the intervertebral disc space. There is currently no universally accepted method for describing such changes, and each institution is often slightly different in this regard. It is also relatively common for physicians within a given center to report these types of changes in a highly individualized manner. This is a polite way of saying that each doctor thinks she or he is correct, and there is clearly no agreed-upon "correct" way to interpret degenerative disc disease. The terminology in question includes *bulge, protrusion, extrusion, herniation,* and *free fragment.*

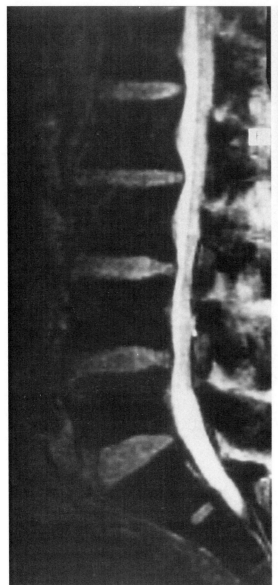

A

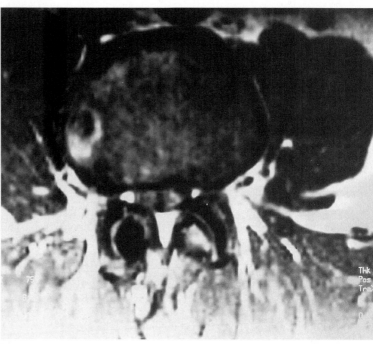

B

Figure 16-5 *A.* Sagittal GRE T2-weighted MR (TR 450, TE 12, FA 12) demonstrating narrowing of the spinal canal secondary to spinal stenosis (compare to *B*). *B.* Axial SE T1-weighted MR (TR 750, TE 15) demonstrating marked narrowing of the spinal canal due to a combination of early osteophyte formation, intervertebral disc bulge, facet hypertrophy, ligamentum flavum enlargement, epidural lipomatosis, and short pedicles.

The term *bulging disc,* or *disc bulge,* generally refers to a condition in which the margins of the intervertebral disc (defined anatomically as the anulus of the disc) remain intact, but are weakened. This laxity in the "disc wall" (anulus) results in a bulging of the disc outside the normal confines of the intervertebral disc space. This has been likened to a jelly doughnut in which the jelly is pushing out against the sides of the doughnut, but the sides have not been ruptured. This will generally be seen on the MRI as the intervertebral disc bulging, protruding, or sticking out beyond its normal margins in a relatively smooth and uniform fashion (see Fig. 16-9*A* and *B*). By definition, there can be no "focal" component to a disc bulge.

The term *intervertebral disc protrusion* is sometimes used as synonymous with a disc herniation. However, it is the degree of "focal" change that determines whether the protruding disc is bulging or herniated. This can be a confusing point, and often a disc that is bulging to one observer is protruding to another. Sometimes the observer will simply use the term *disc protrusion* to indicate that she or he is not certain whether the disc is actually ruptured.

One of the more common and severe complications of degenerative spine disease is actual disc herniation, also referred to as disc rupture or herniated nucleus pulposis (HNP). Exclusion of this finding is often the clinical description given at the time the MRI of the spine is requested, leading to the frequently encountered request form with the designation "R/O HNP" (meaning "rule out herniated nucleus pulposis") or "R/O DISC" (meaning "rule out ruptured disc"). MRI is generally the preferred

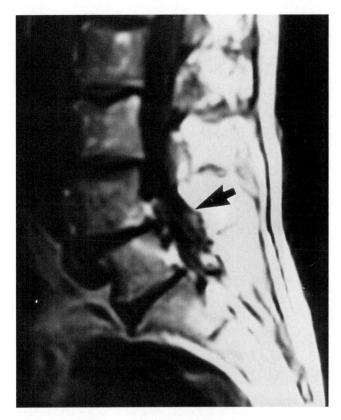

Figure 16-6 Sagittal SE T1-weighted MR (TR 438, TE 20) demonstrating the appearance of a grade I spondylolisthesis at L4-L5 *(arrow)*. Note how the vertebral body of L4 is projecting anteriorly over the vertebral body of L5. (Compare to Fig. 16-7.)

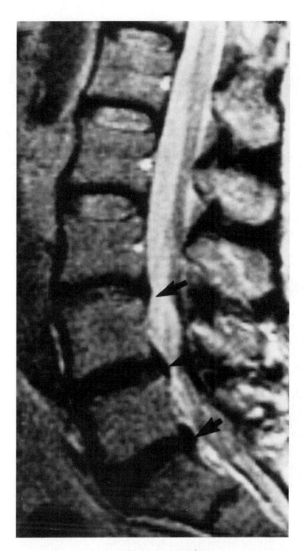

Figure 16-8 Sagittal SE T2-weighted MR (TR 2000, TE 80) demonstrating disc bulges and loss of intervertebral disc signal due to degeneration *(arrows)*. (Compare to the normal disc signal in the higher-level intervertebral discs on this exam.)

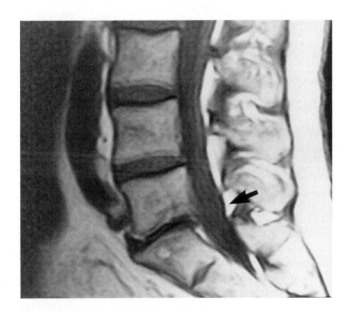

Figure 16-7 Sagittal SE T1-weighted MR (TR 500, TE 20) demonstrating the appearance of a retrolisthesis at L5-S1 *(arrow)*. Note how the vertebral body of L5 is projecting posteriorly over the vertebral body of S1. (Compare to Fig. 16-6.)

method for the evaluation of a possible ruptured disc, and changes and disc disruption are readily identified on MRI. Degeneration of the intervertebral disc is often encountered in the absence of disc herniation (see Fig. 16-8); however, it is uncommon to see disc rupture without evidence of disc degeneration. This is particularly true of ruptured lumbar discs, and most disc herniations do occur in the lumbar region (see Fig. 16-10*A* and *B*). An exception is acute traumatic disc rupture such as occurs with spine trauma from falls or automobile accidents.

A very important finding that may or may not accompany intervertebral disc rupture is that of a *free fragment*. This finding can be overlooked, and the alert technologist can point it out when it is present in association with a ruptured intervertebral disc. Essentially what has occurred in the case of a free fragment is that a piece of the disc material has separated from the main component and

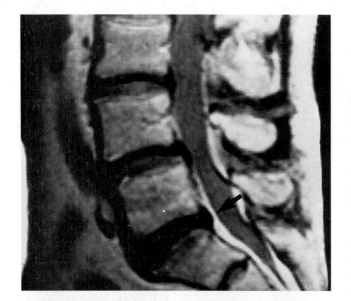

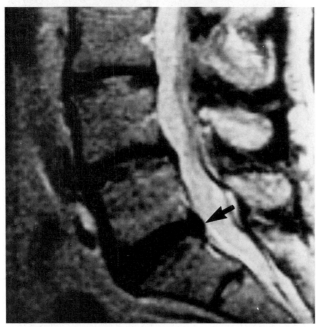

Figure 16-9 *A.* Sagittal SE proton-density-weighted MR (TR 2000, TE 30) demonstrating a prominent intervertebral disc bulge at L5-S1 *(arrow)* (compare to *B*). *B.* Sagittal SE T2-weighted MR (TR 2000, TE 80) demonstrating a disc bulge and loss of intervertebral disc signal due to degeneration *(arrow)* (compare to *A*).

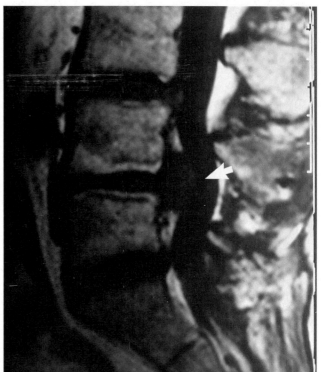

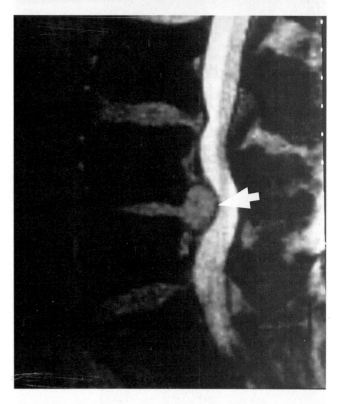

Figure 16-10 *A.* Sagittal SE T1-weighted MR (TR 500, TE 15) demonstrating a large herniated disc at L4-L5 *(arrow)*. Note that there is also narrowing of the intervertebral disc space at this level (compare to *B*). *B.* Sagittal GRE T2-weighted MR (TR 450, TE 12, FA 12) demonstrating narrowing of the interverte-bral disc space at L4-L5 with an associated large herniated disc *(arrow)* (compare to *A*).

has moved away. This free fragment of disc material is within the spinal canal, but often located away from the usual intervertebral disc level. Another term for the free fragment is *sequestered disc.* Most of the time, the free fragment or sequestered disc material will move laterally (to one side) and will compress a nerve root. However, this may be well above or below the level of the disc herniation (see Fig. 16-11).

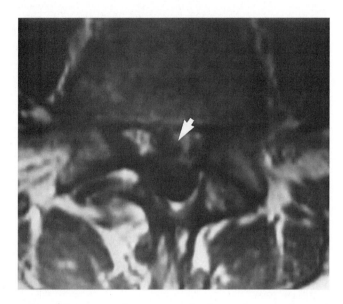

Figure 16-11 Axial SE T1-weighted MR (TR 800, TE 15) demonstrating a free disc fragment *(arrow)* resulting in narrowing of the spinal canal and nerve root compression.

A patient study that is difficult to interpret and often equally difficult for the technologist to perform is that of the postoperative spine. Following spinal surgery, the normal anatomy of the spine can be significantly altered, and the MRI may be extremely difficult to interpret. In addition to the tissue disruption caused by the surgical incision, there may also be metallic artifacts on the MRI from clips, staples, or filings from drills used in the surgical procedure. In the lumbar postoperative spine, gadolinium contrast is generally utilized. However, contrast is of less benefit in the postoperative cervical or thoracic spine study unless there is concern for infection or tumor.

The technique for performing a contrast-enhanced MRI of the spine, particularly in the postoperative patient, is more demanding than routine imaging, and the technologist must be careful when doing this study. It is extremely important that comparable images for both precontrast and postcontrast sequences be obtained. Therefore, it is imperative that the patient remain in the exact same position for both precontrast and postcontrast scans. Starting an IV or heparin lock before imaging patients with a history of prior surgery, then injecting them following the noncontrasted scan minimizes the chance that the patient's position will change between scans. If it is necessary to remove the patient from a bore type of scanner after the noncontrasted scan in order to perform the injection, then the patient must be returned to the same position (or as close as possible) following the infusion of contrast.

In addition to obtaining scans in the sagittal and axial planes before and after contrast, it is also necessary to complete the postcontrast examination within approxi-

mately 20 minutes of the injection. When a lower-field-strength scanner is used, the imaging times may be prolonged, and a constant drip infusion of gadolinium or a double or triple dose may be of benefit. One method of providing prolonged contrast enhancement for the longer scan times that are frequently encountered at lower field strengths is to bolus half of the dose of gadolinium and then to drip-infuse the completion of the scan. The gadolinium can be diluted in normal saline if necessary; however, if any other type of solution is used (such as a glucose solution), caution must be taken to avoid any type of precipitate. One of the most common reasons to perform the gadolinium scan following surgery is to differentiate scar tissue from recurrent disc herniation.

Although an MRI scan without and with gadolinium contrast enhancement six weeks or more after surgery is currently one of the most effective ways of evaluating the postoperative spine, this procedure may be fraught with difficulty. Scar tissue should normally enhance and residual or recurrent disc material should normally remain unenhanced, giving a significant tissue signal difference. However, a small amount of disc material may be "lost"

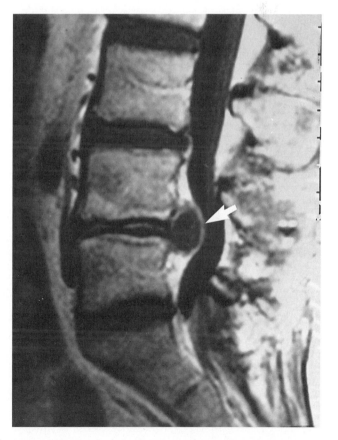

Figure 16-12 Sagittal SE T1-weighted MR (TR 500, TE 15) after administration of gadolinium demonstrating a large herniated disc at L4-L5 *(arrow).* Note that there is narrowing of the intervertebral disc space at this level as well as surrounding contrast enhancement. (Compare to Fig. 16-10.)

when there is a large amount of scar, particularly when partial volume averaging occurs. In addition, scar tissue can actually invade the disc, causing it to enhance and thus obscuring the disc material. Nonetheless, the contrast-enhanced scan viewed with the noncontrast examination at the same levels remains the overall best way to exclude residual or recurrent disc material following surgery (see Fig. 16-12).

Some authors prefer to use the term *disc protrusion* for all forms of intervertebral disc extension beyond the normal confines of the intervertebral disc space. This type of classification would lead to degrees of disc protrusion, commonly referred to as mild, moderate, or severe. These observers would then qualify the study to include a focal component (usually indicating disc rupture) or a sequestered disc when appropriate. In reality, virtually every combination of terminology is used in the interpretation of degenerative disc disease. The final MRI report will usually reflect a combination of the observer's training and experience and the referring clinician's level of understanding. Regardless of the reporting method utilized, the findings of the MRI studies are the same, and with only a little effort, the MRI technologist can readily identify any or all of them.

Suggested Reading

Orrison WW Jr: *Introduction to Neuroimaging.* Boston, Little Brown, 1989.

17

Musculoskeletal Imaging

MRI has added a new dimension to the evaluation of the extremities of the musculoskeletal system. It is considered to be the most sensitive noninvasive imaging method for evaluating a broad spectrum of disease processes affecting the musculoskeletal system. It has enabled us to directly observe structures of the body, such as tendons and ligaments, muscles, and bone marrow, that were not detectable by any other imaging technique. MRI's high contrast resolution can be used to differentiate body tissues and pathology, increasing diagnostic sensitivity and accuracy. Conventional radiography, such as projection and CT radiography, may be helpful in detecting gross bony fractures or destruction of bone; however, the anatomical association of the disease and the extent of the process can be assessed with confidence using high-resolution MRI.

General Considerations

In all cases of musculoskeletal imaging, a combination of T1- and T2-weighted and proton-density images in at least two planes is required to evaluate the area. For evaluation of a mass, the entire compartment of the mass must be seen. Fields of view just large enough to cover the mass area and surrounding anatomy should be chosen. In selected situations, gadolinium injection, gradient echo images, and/or STIR images may be beneficial. When gadolinium injection is indicated, pre- and postcontrast scans should be performed in more than one plane. The

use of intraarticular gadolinium injection may prove helpful in the evaluation of the knee and shoulder.[1] Kinematic and dynamic imaging of the knee and shoulder may also prove beneficial. When the images obtained are visualized using a cine loop, range of motion (kinematic) and functional aspects of the muscles and joints (dynamic) can be evaluated. Very short acquisition times, primarily via the use of gradient echo techniques along with coils designed to allow movement of the extremity are necessary for successful kinematic or dynamic imaging.

The musculoskeletal system of the extremities is small when compared to other anatomic regions of the body such as the head and spine. Therefore, in order to obtain image quality consistent with high-resolution images, scan parameters that affect the voxel volume (FOV, matrix, pixel size, and slice thickness) that are small enough to match the anatomy should be chosen. Except with bilateral imaging of the hip, FOVs between 10 and 20 cm, pixel dimensions less than 1 mm, and a slice thickness less than 5 mm provide the best spatial resolution for musculoskeletal imaging. Matrices can generally be reduced because of the smaller FOVs that are commonly used, thus reducing scan time while maintaining high resolution.

Physiological motion such as flow and respirations can affect the quality of images of the musculoskeletal region. Except for shoulder imaging, this is not a significant source of artifacts. However, even a small amount of flow artifact, such as that seen in axial elbow imaging, can degrade the images. The use of artifact-suppression techniques such as presaturation, flow compensation, and antialiasing can greatly improve the quality of images of these regions and should be considered. When selecting techniques to minimize flow, it is necessary to consider the direction of predominant flow and target the technique (e.g., apply presaturation bands or flow compensation in the superior-inferior direction of the elbow) in the direction that will be most beneficial. Refer to Chap. 12 for a descriptive guide to these applications. Antialiasing techniques can be used to help eliminate wraparound, flow artifacts, and respiratory artifacts. This is done by selectively reconstructing only the area within the display matrix which *should* be the anatomy of interest. Any areas outside this display matrix or within the acquisition matrix will be ignored, thus eliminating any signal that might contribute to an artifact.

Because of the lateral nature of the extremities relative to the isocenter of the magnet, special attention must be paid when performing scout or locator images using a small or midrange FOV. This avoids possible confusion in right-left labeling that may occur in selected cases. Unlike the readout and (2D) slice select dimensions, the phase-encoding dimension in MRI does not distinguish left from right, or head from feet, or anterior from posterior. Images alias every 360 degrees: Left becomes/is right and right becomes/is left. For a symmetric phantom, there can be confusion for any PE direction. In human imaging, the confusion affects only (or mostly) the left-right direction, since the anatomy will always say something about itself in the cases of head-feet or anterior-posterior, even with some PE aliasing.

Mistakes can occur in right-left labeling when a scout image of an extremity has been acquired using a small field of view. The resultant image can be labeled incorrectly if (a) the anatomy aliases on itself *and* (b) the operator uses a portion of the image that appears on the opposite side of the display screen from its true anatomic labeling to plan subsequent images. An example: The right hand is imaged for a locator scan using a small FOV. The hand aliases, so that a portion of the hand is displayed on the right side of the screen while another portion is displayed on the left side of the screen, which is labeled. The operator scrolls the image displayed on the left to the center and plans for subsequent scans from this portion of the hand. The resultant images appear as if the hand that was imaged is from the wrong side (i.e., it is labeled "left" now).

To avoid mistakes such as the above example, some special precautions should be taken.

1. Always use a PE FOV large enough to prevent PE aliasing, which may cause left-right confusion.
2. If a small FOV is selected, measure or estimate an offset along the PE direction of the extremity for use in performing the locator scan. For example, an average-size woman's shoulder is approximately 160 mm from the magnet isocenter. This can be used as the electronic offset so that the shoulder image is approximately in the center of the display screen.
3. If aliasing does occur because both 1 and 2 are violated (by accident or by choice), relate reality to the labeling and planning to avoid mistakes. For example, use the

portion of the labeled anatomy of the graphical locator to match reality in scan planning.

Coil selection is critical in obtaining optimal tissue contrast and definition of the small body parts normally associated with the musculoskeletal system. SNR is related to the size of the coil, so that when coil size is large, coverage is increased, but at a cost of an increase in both signal *and* noise.[2] An improvement in the SNR can be realized by placing the anatomical region as close to the coil antenna as possible. This assures that the maximum amount of signal from the excited tissue is detected.

Two basic coil configurations are currently used successfully in musculoskeletal imaging: the linear surface coil and the quadrature detection–type coil (QD). Both designs are capable of improving signal-to-noise ratio, and each has advantages and limitations.

Implementation of surface coil technology helps to improve SNR by limiting the area of signal detection, thereby reducing unwanted signal. Surface coils receive signal in an elliptical manner, so that the edge of the coil "sees" less signal than the center of the coil[3] (see Fig. 17-1).

This becomes important, as the signal is dependent on positioning the body part appropriately with respect to the coil. The center of the coil detects the greatest signal, so the body part to be imaged must be placed in this location.

A disadvantage associated with surface coils, however, is related to the increase in signal detection. Since most surface coils currently used to image relatively small anatomic regions are positioned very close to the anatomy, "hot spots" of signal can be seen in areas of increased fat. This can be corrected by incorporating a small amount of distance between the coil and the body part (e.g., padding with a very small piece of foam) so that the signal from the fat, as detected by the coil, actually diminishes somewhat because it is farther from the coil. A word of caution: Too much distance between the coil and the body part can decrease the overall signal unnecessarily by pushing the area of interest out of the sensitive detection area of the coil. Some manufacturers have reconstruction pro-

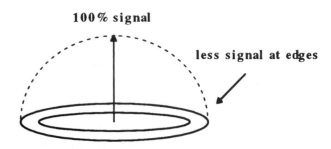

Figure 17-1 Surface coil with elliptical-shape signal reception. Within the radius of the coil, 100 percent signal is detected; signal drops off at the edges of the coil.

grams that attenuate this excessively bright signal associated with surface coil imaging so that it does not appear as such.

Small surface coils are commonly quite flexible and can be positioned in many different ways. That is, they can be maneuvered to fit the body part because they generally are not fixed to a coil base which must be attached to the table in a specific manner. An important rule that pertains to coil technology must be followed to ensure optimum signal detection: The coil must be positioned so that the receive path of the coil (the transverse magnetization plane) is perpendicular to the main magnetic field, $β_0$ or longitudinal magnetization. The coil will produce the strongest signal when the transverse magnetization is aligned with the polarization direction of the coil. When the transverse magnetization vector rotates in and out of the receive coil, a current is produced. The stronger the magnetization, the stronger the current and the greater the detected signal.[4] Since our transmitter is really the excited tissue, which has a rotating magnetic field associated with the oscillating frequency, the strongest signal will be obtained when the magnetization vector is at 90° or 270° to the main field when using linear-type coils. If the receive coil is positioned at an angle, transverse magnetization is not affecting the antenna adequately, so that less current is induced in the coil, resulting in a reduction of detected signal. When positioning surface coils about body parts, it is important to remember to orient the receive path of the coil so that it is perpendicular to the main magnetic field. This orientation will result in the strongest and most consistent signal production. Check with the manufacturer for the specifics of the coil to determine proper orientation.

Quadrature coil design improves SNR significantly by detecting the signal in a circularly polarized manner, much like rotation of the magnetic field vector. The rotating magnetic field of the tissues is forced to move in and out of the xy plane as a result of resonance. Linear coil technology, used in surface coil imaging, detects the signal in only one plane, even though the tissue transmitter is circularly polarized. Quadrature technology uses two channels whose coils receive a signal from phases that are offset from one another by 90°. The two signals are electronically added, providing an improvement in SNR of approximately 41 percent (square root of 2).[5] This is, of course, the advantage of quadrature detection. As this is coupled with the small relative size of the QD extremity coil, SNR for small body parts is usually quite good.

Quadrature coils used in extremity imaging are usually fixed to a coil base (many look like small versions of QD head coils) and can be positioned on the table in only one orientation. This results in the need to maneuver the patient's body part to fit the coil, which may prove difficult in some instances. The extremity being examined must be centrally placed in the coil to ensure maximum and homogeneous signal detection. Many times this requires "creative padding" techniques. If the extremity is very small, clipping can result because the RF power level and receiver gain values are not appropriately chosen during the coil tuning. If the system allows it, lowering the receiver gain by several decibels can help reduce this error (see Chap. 6, "Artifacts").

General rules regarding the efficiency of coils are as follows:

1. The smaller the coil, the better the SNR. Match the coil size to the body part.
2. Match the selected FOV to the coil size and anatomic region of interest.
3. Quadrature coils tend to yield images with better SNR than surface coils, but this can be dependent on the size of the body part being imaged. For instance, when imaging a toe or a finger, the smallest surface coil available (i.e., 100-mm coil) may be a better choice than a QD extremity coil, since the QD coil may be much larger than the area of interest.
4. Choose a coil that will allow the most patient comfort. Any potential improvement in image quality gained by selecting a particular coil can be lost if a patient is uncomfortable.

Soft Tissue

The excellent soft tissue characterization afforded by MR imaging has proved highly beneficial in the evaluation of a variety of soft tissue injuries and diseases. When fat-suppression techniques are added to the imaging repertoire, diagnostic accuracy can be greatly improved. Table 17-1 identifies various clinical indications for which MRI is useful in the evaluation of soft tissue abnormalities.

TABLE 17-1 CLINICAL INDICATIONS— SOFT TISSUE

Traumatic injuries of muscle, tendons, and ligaments
Hematomas
Compartment syndromes
Entrapment syndromes
Tendinosis
Tenosynovitis
Bursitis
Infections and abscesses
Myositis
Cysts (nonneoplastic, parameniscal, and ganglion types)
Detection, staging, and characterization of neoplasms

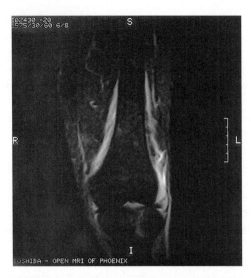

Figure 17-2 Coronal STIR image of knee shows fracture through tibial plateau. *(Courtesy Open MRI of Phoenix. By permission.)*

Bones

Most bone pathology can be defined using short T1-weighted, proton-density, and T2-weighted imaging techniques. However, subtle injuries, infections, and infiltrative diseases are better seen using fat-suppression techniques, such as STIR (see Fig. 17-2).

A variety of bone tumors can be well seen using MRI. They include tumors arising from the bone and cartilage, connective tissue, fibrohistiocytic and hematopoietic origins, and plasma cells. Miscellaneous tumors arising from processes such as aneurysmal bone cysts and Gaucher's disease can be well seen using MR imaging techniques. A partial list of bone abnormalities that can be evaluated using MRI is given in Table 17-2.

TABLE 17-2 CLINICAL INDICATIONS—BONE

Traumatic injury to bone; occult injury of the metaphysis and epiphysis
Evaluation of bone fracture union
Osteomyelitis
Periprosthetic infections
Detection and staging of primary bone tumors and bony metastases
Detection and extent of congenital lesions (fibrous dysplasia and C1-C2 abnormalities)
Osteonecrosis and bone infarcts
Avascular necrosis

Joints

The evaluation of joints has historically been accomplished using conventional radiographic techniques in the form of arthrography. These imaging methods require the intraarticular injection of radio-opaque contrast media and the physical manipulation of the joint by either the radiologist or the technologist. In most cases, this is quite painful for the patient. Radiation exposure is also an added, well-documented risk, although the risk is not as significant as it was in the early days of x-ray technology. Using magnetic resonance imaging techniques, joints can be evaluated in any plane or variant thereof, without the use of contrast agents, radiation exposure, or stress maneuvers. Pulse sequence protocols can be designed to provide sufficient contrast to evaluate the joint and associated structures. Although injection of gadolinium into a joint is advocated by some investigators, it is not the usual protocol, so that joint evaluation using MRI continues to be a noninvasive diagnostic procedure. Dynamic and/or kinematic imaging techniques can be used to assess the function of structures surrounding the joint. Imaging planes can be selected to coincide with the primary axes of the structures being evaluated. Basically, a three-dimensional assessment of the area can be provided without unnecessary pain and suffering to the patient. Table 17-3 lists various clinical indications for which MRI is useful.

Shoulder Imaging

The shoulder is susceptible to a good deal of mechanical stress and strain during our lives. Pain is common and

TABLE 17-3 CLINICAL INDICATIONS—JOINTS

Traumatic injuries to joints and surrounding muscle, tendons, and ligaments
Articular cartilage injuries
Bursitis
Synovitis
Fragment instability
Cartilage status in osteochondritis dissecans
Degenerative joint disease
Loose bodies
Tenosynovitis
Joint infections
Rheumatoid and the seronegative arthritides
Overuse synovitis
Ganglion and bursal cysts
Abscesses
Benign and malignant neoplasms
Avascular necrosis of associated bone
Degenerative joint disease

sometimes debilitating. The upper extremity, including the neck, is constantly involved in motion requiring heavy weight bearing, the use of force, and complex movements. Soft tissues of the region include nerves, blood vessels, muscles, ligaments, and tendons which are compressed into tight compartments. Injury to this region is quite common.

The bony configuration of the shoulder girdle comprises the head of the humerus, the scapula, which includes the rim of the glenoid cavity, the coracoid process and the acromion, and the clavicle. The acromioclavicular joint is the most superior aspect of the shoulder. The ball-and-socket-type shoulder joint has the greatest freedom of movement of any joint in the body. Even though the bony configuration results in a mobile joint, it is inherently unstable. The presence of an articular cuff made up of muscles and tendons, known as the "rotator cuff," greatly strengthens the joint except inferiorly, where dislocations frequently occur. The muscles include the supraspinatus, infraspinatus, and subscapularis and their tendons, and the tendon of the teres minor. Working as a group, they hold the head of the humerus in the glenoid fossa. The tendons can be seen as a homogeneous very low (black) signal on MRI (see Fig. 17-3). The musculature of the shoulder region provides for abduction, adduction, rotation, flexion, and extension of the upper extremity and is depicted in Table 17-4.

The major nerves that supply the shoulder originate from the brachial plexus. They are the axillary, suprascapular, and subscapular nerves. These nerves innervate the muscles that provide for movement of our upper extremities. Damage to the nerve itself, to any portion of the brachial plexus, or to the ventral rami of the fifth through eight cervical and first thoracic nerves (from which the brachial plexus originates) may produce symptoms in the shoulder region.

Vascular supply to the shoulder is derived from various branches of the axillary artery. The thoracoacromial artery branches to supply the clavicle, the acromion process, and the deltoid muscle. The humeral circumflex provides vascularity to the anterior and posterior portions of the humerus. The subscapular artery sends branches to the musculature of the scapula via the scapular circumflex artery and the thoracodorsal branch.

Pathologic processes producing symptoms may be local or may be distant, causing radiation of pain along the neurovascular bundles anywhere from the spinal cord to the end of the extremity, or may be derived from intrathoracic or upper abdominal structures. Symptoms can be a result of inflammation, pain, motion limitation, weakness, muscle atrophy, or a mass. It is important to obtain a thorough history of the patient's complaint so that the imaging procedure can be tailored to the clinical findings.

Evaluation of the shoulder joint and associated structures is commonly performed using MRI. MRI is indicated for pain of undetermined etiology, detection and staging of rotator cuff degeneration and tears, impingement syndromes, labral degenerative changes and tears, biceps tendon disease and dislocation, suprascapular notch syndrome, glenohumeral ligament injuries, coracoclavicular and acromioclavicular separations, subacromial bursitis, and postfracture assessment. It is the best imaging procedure for evaluating the sources of impingement in a completely noninvasive manner. MRI can reliably assess bone marrow as well as soft tissue processes such as lipomas or muscular tears. In some instances, intraarticular contrast administration may be warranted to better detect labral tears and/or instability. This can be accomplished using MRI after gadolinium or saline injection or by CT arthrography.[6]

The imaging plane should be chosen to coincide with the primary axes of the shoulder and to display the true shape and contour of the shoulder anatomy. The planes should include axial, oblique coronal, and oblique sagittal. A common approach to scanning the shoulder is to provide oblique orientation of the shoulder, either electronically or by positioning the patient in a coronal orientation. A posterior oblique orientation of approximately 15 to 30° (posterior affected side down) can be achieved by using positioning sponges to prop the patient, much like positioning for an oblique x-ray of the lumbar spine. This also allows a more natural external rotation of the arm, which is necessary for adequate visualization of separate structures. Electronic obliquity is easily performed; however, as a result of the process of producing an oblique from two orthogonal planes (two slice select gradient functions are required), the image quality may not be as good as that achieved by physically positioning the patient and

TABLE 17-4 MUSCLES OF THE SHOULDER

Abductors	Adductors	Rotators	Flexion/Extension	Rotator Cuff
Deltoideus	Teres major	Infraspinatus	Subscapularis	Supraspinatus *m/t*
Supraspinatus	Teres minor	Subscapularis	Deltoideus	Infraspinatus *m/t*
Subscapularis	Subscapularis	Deltoideus		Supscapularis *m/t*
		Teres major		Teres minor *t*

m = muscle and *t* = tendon in denoting the muscles and tendons that make up the rotator cuff.

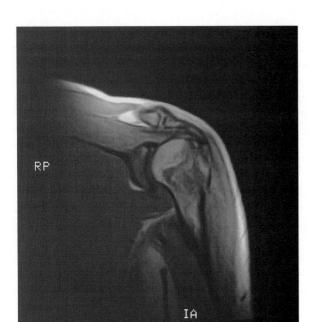

Figure 17-3 Off-coronal image of shoulder. *(Courtesy Open MRI of Phoenix. By permission.)*

performing an orthogonal-type acquisition. This is of course true for any electronically obliqued acquisition. In either case, slices that are parallel to the supraspinatus muscle or perpendicular to the glenoid fossa of the scapula should be obtained. This ensures that the supraspinatus muscle and the other components of the rotator cuff and glenoid labrum are well seen. The patient should be positioned in somewhat of an external rotation for the oblique coronal, as internal rotation creates an overlap of the supraspinatus and infraspinatus tendons.

For axial and oblique sagittal imaging, a "thumbs up" or neutral orientation is sufficient.[7]

As MR technology has improved, several modifications in shoulder imaging techniques have been seen. There is a general consensus among clinicians that protocols selected for evaluating the shoulder should include a combination of T1, T2 or proton-density, and gradient echo images. One approach to examining the shoulder is given in Table 17-5.

When soft tissue pathology, lipoma, or bone marrow disease is suspected, a fat-suppression sequence such as STIR is beneficial in defining the location and extent of the process.

Most pathology of the shoulder involves the center of the supraspinatus musculotendinous complex. Impingement syndrome is claimed to be the precursor to rotator cuff injuries in 95 percent of cases. It commonly results from entrapment of the supraspinatus tendon between the humeral head and the inferior portion of the acromion clavicle (AC) joint capsule. Causes may include spurring below the AC joint, fibrous thickening of the AC joint capsule or ligament, a low-lying acromion process, or hypertrophy of the supraspinatus muscle. These may be a result of previous trauma to the shoulder region, arthritis, or well-developed musculature in healthy individuals.

Any overgrowth of the AC joint, either fibrous or bony, may impinge inferiorly on the musculotendinous junction of the supraspinatus. A low-lying acromion, which normally should fall within boundaries established by drawing a subclavicular line, can also cause impingement syndrome. This may be identified by observing a deviation of the normal fat stripe which runs along the inferior surface of the clavicle, acromion, and deltoid muscle. This fat stripe has a normal diameter of approximately

TABLE 17-5 REPRESENTATION OF IMAGING PLANES FOR SHOULDER ASSESSMENT

Plane	Sequence	Structures Assessed	Positioning
Axial	T1, PD, T2 or T2°	Supraspinatus and associated structures, glenoid labrum, other rotator cuff structures. T2° good for assessing fluids.	Perpendicular to off-coronal plane.
Oblique sagittal	T1, PD, or T2	Anterior acromion and AC joint relative to rotator cuff, subacromial space.	Perpendicular to off-coronal plane or long axis of body of scapula.
Oblique coronal	T1	Marrow signal and fat stripe, rotator cuff, ACJ, glenoid labrum, continuous view of supraspinatus tendon.	Parallel to long axis of body of scapula or supraspinatus muscle. Perpendicular to glenoid fossa.

2 mm. Athletes such as swimmers and weight lifters, who tend to have hypertrophied supraspinatus muscles, may also manifest the impingement syndrome because of the muscle taking space that normally would be occupied by the fat stripe.

The MR appearance of the shoulder region is well demonstrated. The musculotendinous junction of the supraspinatus is well seen, with the tendon appearing darker than the muscle (see Fig. 17-3). If a defect exists, fluid will fill the defect and appear bright on a T2-weighted image. Nonvisualization of fluid does not preclude a tear, however. The muscle is normally homogeneous with relatively low signal; it is fusiform in shape. Higher signal intensity may indicate scarring, edema, inflammation, or other abnormal condition. With longstanding impingement, there is loss of muscle volume and an increased signal intensity. The appearance of a bright signal between the supraspinatus and infraspinatus muscles may indicate normally situated fat. The ligaments of the shoulder include the acromioclavicular, coraco-clavicular, coraco-acromio, and coraco-humeral. They can be difficult to identify because of their similarity in appearance to a filling defect on MRI but can be observed on sequential slices as dark-appearing structures.

Bone marrow is readily seen with MRI. It should not be overlooked as the source of patient symptoms, as it is a prime site for avascular necrosis, metastatic disease, primary tumors, and bone cysts. In addition, preservation of the red marrow in the metaphyseal region may be identified. At birth, all the marrow throughout the skeleton is active and is virtually the sole source of blood cells. By adult life, over one-half of the bone marrow has been replaced by yellow or fatty marrow, which is hematopoietically inactive. In some cases, hematopoiesis is reinitiated by the body's need for red cells, so that fatty marrow is transformed to active, red marrow. This can be differentiated from metastatic disease by performing a T1-weighted image on the contralateral side or by observing an intermediate signal intensity on T1, proton-density, and T2 sequences.[8]

Elbow Imaging

Most elbow injuries are a result of overuse rather than acute trauma. This chronic stress and repetitive microtrauma such as is experienced by quarterbacks, pitchers, and golfers may be difficult to diagnose. Although no standard for MRI of elbow imaging has been described, the procedure is extremely useful for evaluating inflammation of tendons and muscles, bone marrow, and cartilaginous abnormalities. Because of MRI's excellent tissue contrast, other soft tissue lesions such as ganglion cysts, neuromas, hematomas, and lipomas are also well seen.

The elbow is a difficult extremity to image because of

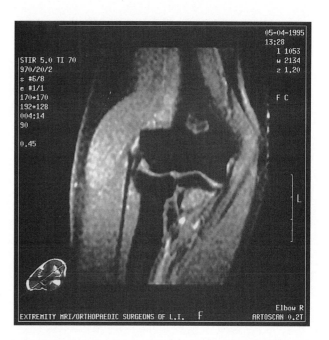

Figure 17-4 Elbow image obtained on 0.2-T permanent extremity magnet. *(Courtesy of LUNAR Corporation. By permission.)*

its anatomical relationship to the body, which is longitudinally placed in the magnet. The difficulty involves positioning the elbow, taking into account coil criteria, the lateral aspect of the extremity with regard to magnet isocenter, and patient comfort. Some manufacturers address this difficulty by allowing only the extremity to be placed in the isocenter of the magnet. The patient is positioned on a reclining chair outside the magnet, with the extremity of interest extending into the bore. The extremity can be positioned in the small FOV receiver coil in anatomical orientation (see Fig. 17-4).

The elbow should be imaged while at the patient's side, whenever possible, when using conventional MR imagers. This position is ideal with regard to patient comfort and true anatomic orientation. Surface coil imaging works best, since the coil can be maneuvered to accommodate the placement of the elbow. The smallest coil available that will cover the anatomy and provide the most patient comfort should be used. FOVs that match the coil size will result in the best resolution and minimize the potential for aliasing. T1 and T2 contrast images should be obtained, using slice thicknesses that correspond to the small anatomy associated with the elbow (generally less than 4 mm). STIR imaging is recommended when there is a question of tear, bone marrow disease, or soft tissue infection. In some cases, saline MR arthrography may provide detailed information regarding the presence of intraarticular loose bodies, when joint effusion is not present (see Fig. 17-5).[9]

Table 17-6 identifies the common anatomical struc-

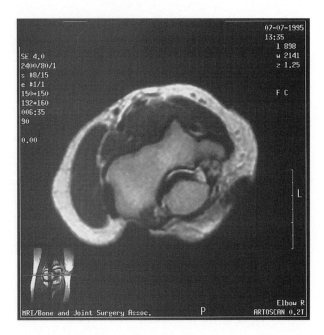

Figure 17-5 T2 axial elbow image. (*Courtesy LUNAR Corporation. By permission.*)

tures contained in the elbow region and the imaging plane in which they can be well visualized using MRI.

Hand, Wrist, and Finger Imaging

MRI is indicated for evaluation of tendon and ligamentous injuries, injury to the triangular fibrocartilage, extensor and flexor tenosynovitis, carpal tunnel syndrome, and soft tissue processes such as hemangiomas, tendon sheath cysts, ganglions, and lipomas. MRI is highly useful for detecting and localizing avascular necrosis, commonly associated with navicular fractures (see Fig. 17-6).

Distal upper extremity imaging involves the same difficulty as elbow imaging because of the lateral orientation of the extremity with respect to the magnet isocenter. It is essential to use small surface coils for imaging the distal upper extremity, as they are much easier to position and provide high-resolution images with minimal artifacts from extraneous noise.

Imaging planes should be carefully chosen to corre-

TABLE 17-6 COMMON ANATOMICAL STRUCTURES OF THE ELBOW AND ASSOCIATED IMAGING PLANES

Structure	Location or Function	Plane
Tendons/Ligaments		
Biceps tendon	Radial tuberosity insertion	Axial/sagittal
Triceps tendon	Olecranon insertion	Axial/sagittal
Common flexor tendon	Medial/anterior ulna	Axial/coronal
Common extensor tendon	Adjacent to annular ligament	Axial/coronal
Annular ligament	Curves around radial head	Axial
Radial collateral ligament	Lateral epicondyle–annular ligament	Coronal
Medial collateral ligament	Medial epicondyle–ulna	Coronal
Articulations		
Radioulnar	Pivotal joint	Axial
Radial head–capitellar joint	Ball and socket joint (flexion/ extension/pronation/supination)	Sagittal
Trochlear–ulnar articulation	Hinge joint	Sagittal
Soft Tissues		
Biceps	Anterior (flexor)	Axial/sagittal/coronal
Triceps	Posterior (extensor)	Axial/sagittal/coronal
Brachialis	Anterior to radial head (flexor)	Axial
Brachioradialis	Lateral (support)	Axial/sagittal/coronal
Supinator	Medial to brachioradialis about radius	Axial/coronal
Pronator teres	Anterior–medial (support)	Axial
Aconeus	Posterior to radius—lateral to ulna	Axial
Anterior and posterior fat pad		Sagittal
Radial nerve	Anterior between brachioradialis and brachialis	Axial/variable
Ulnar nerve	Posterior to medial epicondyle	Axial
Median nerve	Anterior–medial	Axial/variable

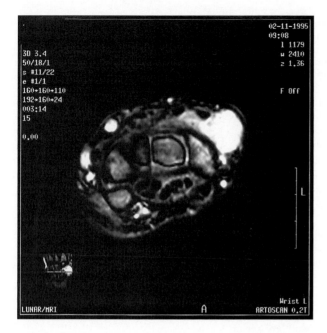

Figure 17-6 Image of hand and wrist. *(Courtesy LUNAR Corporation. By permission.)*

spond to true sagittal, coronal, and axial orientations. An MR-compatible wrist brace may be useful to ensure and maintain proper anatomic alignment. An FOV of 12 cm or less is recommended when using small local surface coils, and slice thickness should be minimal to correspond with the small anatomic region being imaged. 3DFT imaging may improve image quality by increasing the SNR while providing high-resolution images. As in all cases of MR imaging, T1 and T2 sequences are necessary to evaluate all types of pathology. STIR sequences are useful in evaluating bone disease, infections, and the triangular fibrocartilage complex.[10] Table 17-7 identifies the common anatomical structures contained in the hand and wrist and the imaging plane in which they can be well visualized using MRI.

An increasingly common area of wrist imaging is the carpal tunnel region, as this syndrome affects a large portion of the population. The syndrome is a result of narrowing of the canal secondary to trauma, chronic or acute, osteoarthritic changes, and malaligned carpal bones. An increase in the volume of the canal can be associated with (a) growth of tumors such as neuromas, lipomas, hemangiomas, or ganglion cysts; (b) an increase in the normal fat and muscle content of the canal; (c) congenital variations such as persistent median artery; and (d) synovial hypertrophy as seen in rheumatoid arthritis. In any case, compression of the median nerve as a result of canal volume changes produces edema of the nerve, which is readily seen on MRI axial images. When described with an increase in T2 signal, nerve flattening at the level of the pis-

form and distal radius, and a bowed flexor tendon, the MR findings are considered the "sine qua non of carpal tunnel syndrome."[11]

Avascular necrosis (AVN) is readily identified on MR images because of the technique's high sensitivity to marrow signal alterations. AVN is most often seen in the lunate bone following scaphoid fractures (Kienboch disease).

Tears of the triangular fibrocartilage complex (TFC) can be seen on T1 and T2 sequences as high-signal linear bands that extend from one articular surface to another. The majority of TFC tears occur near the ulnar insertion.

MRI continues to have an impact in the evaluation of wrist abnormalities, particularly carpal tunnel syndrome, AVN, triangular fibrocartilage injury, and soft tissue tumors. MRI techniques that provide high-resolution, high-contrast images can be combined with the advantages of surface coil imaging to produce images of exquisite quality (see Fig. 17-7).

Hip Imaging

The primary indication for hip MRI is to rule out early AVN. MRI has been shown thus far to have a very high sensitivity and specificity in this diagnosis, surpassing both bone and CT scanning. It can also be used as an adjunct procedure for evaluating other pathologic conditions of the hip, such as fractures, tumors, infection, degenerative disease, effusion, bursitis, dislocation, and the presence of loose bodies.[12]

Imaging protocols should include T1- and T2-weighted sequences and proton-density images as well as a fat-suppression sequence such as STIR. T1-weighted and STIR coronal images are sensitive for AVN and fractures, whereas T2-weighted images that are of high resolution can provide detailed anatomic information, especially in children (see Fig. 17-8). An FOV large enough to include *both* hips, surrounding soft tissues, and the pelvic girdle is essential for comparative evaluation of symmetry, especially with regard to early AVN. Because of this requirement, most imaging of the hips is performed using volume body coils. Care must be taken to ensure that the patient's body does not touch the coil, as this would cause coupling, resulting in the "hourglass" artifact and aliasing, which degrade image quality.

Table 17-8 identifies the common anatomical structures contained in the hip and the imaging plane in which they can be well visualized using MRI.

AVN, also called *osteonecrosis, aseptic necrosis,* and *ischemic necrosis,* is the bone death process resulting from insufficient blood supply to the subchondral bone in the epiphysis. It can be either nontraumatic or traumatic in origin. The most common site for AVN is in the hip.[13] Traumatic causes such as fracture and/or dislocation commonly result in AVN. Patients with nontraumatic causes of

TABLE 17-7 COMMON ANATOMICAL STRUCTURES OF THE HAND AND WRIST AND ASSOCIATED IMAGING PLANES

Structure	Location or Function	Plane
Tendons/Ligaments		
Scapho-lunate ligament	Scaphoid bone to lunate bone.	Coronal/sagittal
Lunatotriquetral ligaments	Lunate to triquetral bone.	Coronal/sagittal
Flexor tendons	Contained in carpal tunnel with median nerve, palmar surface.	Axial/sagittal
Flexor retinaculum	Sheath extends from pisiform and hook of hamate to scaphoid and trapezium to cover flexor tendons.	Coronal/axial
Extensor tendons	Deep to extensor retinaculum on dorsal surface.	Axial/sagittal
Extensor retinaculum	Sheath extends obliquely from radius to distal ulna, attaching to pisiform and triquetral bone. Covers extensor tendons.	Coronal/axial
Soft Tissues		
Radial nerve	Crosses from anterior forearm to dorsal hand at "anatomic snuff box" region of posterior first metacarpal between tendons.	Axial
Ulnar nerve	Palmar branch is superficial to flexor retinaculum; dorsal branch is cutaneous.	Axial
Median nerve	Carpal tunnel.	Axial
Carpal tunnel	Palmar surface at junction of wrist and forearm. Passageway for tendons and neurovascular structures.	Axial
Bone/Cartilage		
Triangular fibrocartilage	Biconcave band between proximal carpal row and distal ulna/stabilizer.	Coronal/axial
Digits/metacarpals	Thumb–fifth digit.	Sagittal/coronal
Carpal bones	Proximal row: scaphoid, lunate, triquetrum, pisiform. Distal row: trapezium, trapezoid, capitate, hamate.	Coronal
Radius	Lateral.	Axial/coronal/sagittal
Ulna	Medial.	Axial/coronal/sagittal

AVN usually have predisposing conditions, such as sickle cell disease, alcoholism, corticosteroid use, Gaucher's disease, postirradiation, Caisson's disease, gout, or iron overload. It can be idiopathic as well.[14] In some cases, there are no predisposing factors identified.

A classic finding of AVN has been described by Mitchell[15] and consists of a rim of decreased signal intensity on the T1- and T2-weighted images, with an inner band of increased signal intensity seen only on the T2-weighted images. The dark rim is thought to be an area of reactive process between the dead and viable tissue containing inflammatory and fibroblastic tissue and sclerosis due to trabecular bone thickening. Hyperemia in the granulation tissue may provide the bright interzone signal.

MR imaging of the hip is indicated for the evaluation of early AVN because of its proven sensitivity and specificity. It has also proved to be quite useful for the evaluation of metastatic disease, joint effusion, septic joint, and bone abnormalities.

Knee Imaging

The knee is perhaps the most often MR-imaged extremity of the musculoskeletal region. In the past 10 years, MRI has become recognized as a highly accurate diagnostic imaging procedure for a wide variety of knee pathologies. Anatomic knee structures commonly evaluated using MRI

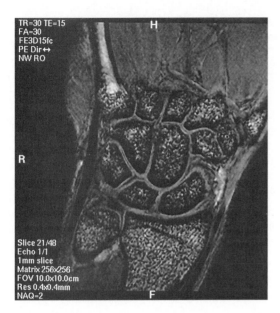

Figure 17-7 Image of hand and wrist. *(Courtesy LUNAR Corporation. By permission.)*

include the menisci, cruciate and collateral ligaments, patellar tendons, and bone marrow. Additionally, vascular lesions, cysts, abnormalities of cartilaginous surfaces, surgical reconstruction and repair, and mass lesions can be assessed with confidence. MRI of the knee provides easily reproducible multiplanar images with high resolution and superb contrast between normal and abnormal tissues (see Fig. 17-9).

The use of dedicated extremity coils, especially of quadrature or phased array design, yields high SNR, which can be "traded" for higher resolution or shorter scan times. Positioning the leg in approximately 15 to 20° external rotation will allow the ACL to be more readily seen in the sagittal plane. All three imaging planes of the knee should be acquired in variations of T1 and T2 or T2* sequences. STIR imaging provides high sensitivity in detecting subtle bone and soft tissue pathology. Slice thicknesses less than 5 mm are preferred, and the smallest FOV with the highest matrix selection that will allow optimum image quality in reasonable scan times is favored. FOVs less than 20 cm and generally closer to 15 cm are the norm. Antialiasing techniques are highly effective in improving image quality (see Chap. 12, "Artifact-Suppression Techniques").

A common filming technique used for MRI of the knee is the "meniscal" window, in which magnified views of the menisci using narrow-contrast windows may increase the detectability of meniscal lesions. This technique is used in addition to the normal filming protocol, in which tears of the menisci are often masked because of the very black appearance of this anatomy.

The important anatomic features of this complex hinge joint are included in Table 17-9.

Pathology commonly seen on MRI includes meniscal and cartilaginous lesions, cruciate and collateral ligament injuries, bony lesions, and cysts. The most common tears of the menisci are the simple oblique vertical and oblique radial tears. Less common tears are those associated with degenerative processes (which appear more horizontal)

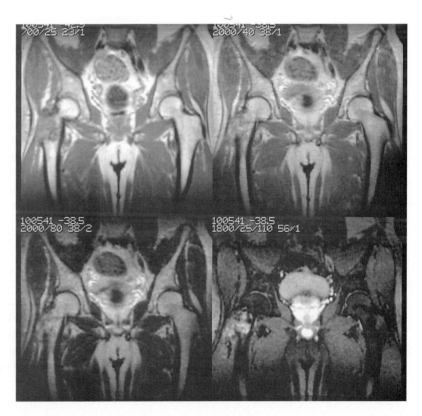

Figure 17-8 T1, T2, and STIR images of the hip. *(Courtesy Toshiba America Medical Systems, Inc. By permission.)*

TABLE 17-8 COMMON ANATOMICAL STRUCTURES OF THE HIP AND ASSOCIATED IMAGING PLANES

Structure	Location or Function	Plane
Bones/Articulation		
Femoral head	Proximal femur.	Coronal/axial
Hip joint	Ball and socket formed by femoral head and acetabulum, covered by cartilage.	Coronal/axial
Fovea capitis	Small depression centrally located on femoral head, attachment site for ligamentum teres.	Coronal/axial
Ligaments/Tendons		
Ligamentum teres	Fovea capitis to acetabulum.	Coronal/axial
Acetabular labrum	Attaches to rim of acetabulum.	Coronal/axial
Muscle Groups		
Posterior	Internal and external obturator, quadratus femoris, piriformis (lateral rotators).	Coronal/axial
Anterior	Quadriceps femoris (extensor).	Axial/sagittal
	Iliopsoas (flexor).	Axial/sagittal
	Sartorius (longest muscle).	Axial/sagittal
Lateral	Gluteus maximus (extensor).	Axial/coronal
	Medius and minimus (medial rotators, abductors).	Axial/coronal
	Tensor fasciae latae (most lateral)	Axial/coronal
Medial	Pectineus, adductors, gracilis (adductors).	Axial/coronal
Neurovascular		
Sciatic nerve	Largest nerve of body (~ 2 cm diameter); posterior to posterior muscle groups and inferolaterally deep to gluteus maximus.	Axial
Femoral artery and vein	Vertically along anteromedial aspect of hip	MRA coronal

bucket handle tears, and peripheral detachments.[16] Tears are classified according to their extension through the meniscus from one articular surface to another, which is seen as an increase in signal on MRI. An increase in signal in the meniscus can also be a result of artifacts such as truncation (low matrix imaging), partial volume (thick-slice imaging), or magic angle (phenomena where connective tissue structures such as tendons and cartilage exhibit a paradoxically low signal if they make an angle of 54.7° with the MR field[17]). In some patients, increased signal within the menisci represents a normal variant from persistent vascularity.

Pseudo tears of the menisci can appear at two common sites: the attachment point between the meniscofemoral ligament and the posteromedial aspect of the lateral meniscus, and the area between the anterior horn of the lateral meniscus and the adjacent transverse meniscal ligament.

Focal areas of cartilaginous thinning associated with repeated trauma to the patella result in the condition chondromalacia patella. Axial images provide helpful information in evaluating this condition.

Cruciate ligament tears can be partial or complete. A sagging appearance or increase in signal with effusion can indicate pathology. However, the thickness and oblique course of the ACL along with variations in signal can give the appearance of a tear when none exists. Secondary signs associated with ACL tears include meniscal tears, bone bruises, anterior displacement of the tibia, and posterior subluxation of the lateral meniscus.[18] When imaging for the collateral ligaments, which are located at the outer surfaces of the knee anatomy, care must be taken to include the entire area. The medial and lateral patellar retinacula and joint capsules are contiguous to the collateral ligaments, and many times cannot be separated from them. A general rule of thumb is to plan slices to cover the medial and lateral edges of the skin when imaging the knee for any reason. This will ensure that all anatomy associated with the knee is adequately included in the image.

**TABLE 17-9 COMMON ANATOMICAL STRUCTURES OF THE HIP
AND ASSOCIATED IMAGING PLANES**

Structure	Location or Function	Plane
Menisci/Cartilage		
Medial and lateral meniscus	Shock absorber between femoral condyles and tibial plateau.	Sagittal
Retropatellar cartilage		Axial
Ligaments/Tendons		
Anterior cruciate	Medial aspect of lateral femoral condyle to anterior tibial spine; prevents anterior displacement of tibia.	Sagittal/axial
Posterior cruciate	Medial femoral condyle to posterior tibia; provides posterior stability to the knee.	Sagittal/axial
Medial and lateral collaterals	Medial: medial femoral condyle to medial tibia (medial support). Lateral: lateral femoral condyle to distal fibular head (lateral support).	Coronal/axial
Meniscofemoral ligament	Anterior, posterior, or both to PCL; superomedial to inferolateral attaching to posterior horn of lateral meniscus.	Sagittal
Quadriceps tendon	Extension of quadriceps femoris muscle group; attaches and surrounds patella, then continues as patellar tendon.	Sagittal
Patellar tendon	Distal quadriceps tendon to tibial tuberosity.	Sagittal
Muscles		
Quadriceps	Anterior muscle group (extensors).	Sagittal/axial
Hamstrings	Posterior muscle group (thigh extensors, leg flexors).	Sagittal/axial
Popliteus	Lateral aspect of lateral femoral condyle to outer margin of lateral meniscus (leg flexor and lateral rotator of femur).	Sagittal/axial
Gastrocnemius	Two-headed, arising from lateral and medial femoral condyles to posterior aspect of knee (leg flexor).	Sagittal/axial
Vascular		
Popliteal artery	Within the popliteal fossa on posterior aspect of knee.	Sagittal

Sources: Mayer DP: MR of the knee. *7th Annual Advances in Mid & Low Field Magnetic Resonance Imaging.* Orlando, FL, September 6–10, 1995. Kelley L, Petersen C: Musculoskeletal imaging, in Bogdan AR, Culbreth LJ (eds): *A Study Guide to MRI. Cross-Sectional Anatomy.* Greenwich, CT. Greenwich Press, 1995.

Fractures of any bony component of the knee are most often identified using conventional x-ray or CT images. However, stress fractures can be more readily detected using MRI because of the associated inflammation processes, which appear dark in signal on T1 images and diffusely bright on T2 and STIR images.[19] The extent of severe fractures and associated soft tissue injury can be assessed as well.

Bone bruises may occur when trauma produces fractures subchondral within the bony trabecula of the marrow without associated cortical involvement (see Fig. 17-10). This is said to have an impact on future shock absorption

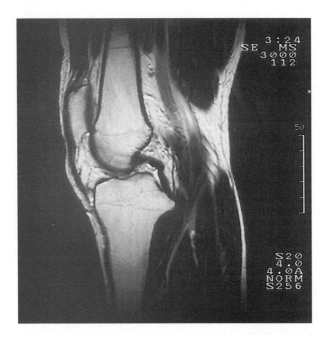

Figure 17-9 Sagittal knee image. (*Courtesy Toshiba America Medical Systems, Inc. By permission.*)

functions of the menisci and cartilage in that they are less able to withstand trauma.[20] Transchondral injuries may result in subsequent AVN, which can be well seen on MRI.

Many types of cysts can be present in the knee. Meniscal cysts associated with tears are common laterally. Synovial cysts contain a gelatinous substance consistent with synovial origin and usually have a connection to the joint capsule as well as the synovial lining. Ganglion cysts, which contain synovial-type cells, necrotic cells, debris, and disintegrated collagen, are subcutaneous lesions about the knee which may or may not communicate with the joint capsule or tendon sheaths.

MRI imaging of the knee has become a highly respected imaging procedure for the evaluation of a wide range of abnormalities. Its reproducibility, absence of ionizing radiation, and noninvasive methods add to the advantages offered by its documented diagnostic accuracy. With the advent of new procedures such as kinematic and dynamic assessment, MR arthrography, and weight-bearing imaging, the technology is sure to increase in popularity.

Foot and Ankle Imaging

The foot and ankle, even though relatively small, are quite complex. They are composed of hinge-type articulations between the tibia, the fibula, and the talus bone that act to plantar- and dorsiflex the extremity. The tarsal bones create a bridge between the lower leg and the metatarsal and phalangeal bones. An architectural web of ligaments and musculotendinous structures within the foot and ankle is oriented in a variety of planes, making identification of specific structures quite challenging.

Although comparative extremity imaging has long been advocated, it is important to perform single-limb imaging when imaging the foot and ankle because of the variations of anatomic angles from ankle to foot and from foot to foot. It is recommended that the extremity to be evaluated be positioned in slight dorsiflexion, with imaging planes oriented as necessary to the area of interest. Optimal imaging includes multiplane imaging of T1, T2, and STIR or other fat-suppression sequences. Fast spin echo imaging techniques and/or rectangular matrices can be used to save scan time while maintaining high contrast and resolution. Scan parameters should be selected to yield high-resolution images and correspond to the small anatomy of interest. FOVs between 10 and 12 cm are opti-

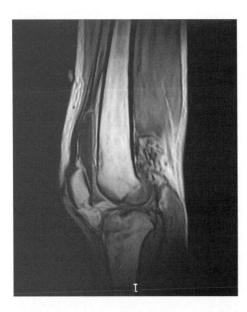

Figure 17-10 Bone contusion and fracture of tibial plateau. (*Courtesy Open MRI of Phoenix. By permission.*)

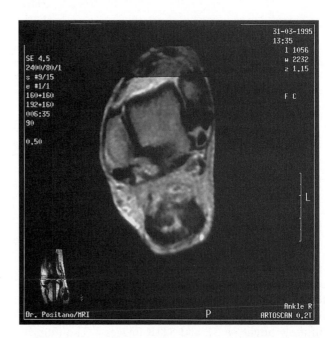

Figure 17-11 Axial ankle image. (*Courtesy LUNAR Corporation. By permission.*)

mal when imaging the forefoot, while 14 to 16 cm can be used for the midfoot and hindfoot. Minimal slice thicknesses are essential for imaging this relatively small region.

When imaging the foot and ankle, it is advisable to consider it as three distinct regions: the hindfoot or ankle, the midfoot, and the forefoot. Ankle imaging should be performed with the ankle as close to 90° (true anatomical orientation) as possible (see Fig. 17-11). Imaging planes should correspond to the specific region being imaged, as the anatomy deviates in orientation from the leg to the tarsals and metatarsals. For example, what is coronal at the level of the hindfoot will be more axial on the mid- and forefoot, relative to anatomic orientation. When imaging joint spaces in the midfoot, planes of section should be oriented through the specific joint spaces. Acquiring images in the midfoot in oblique planes will make interpretation extremely difficult.[21]

Table 17-10 identifies the commonly injured anatomi-

TABLE 17-10 COMMONLY INJURED ANATOMY OF THE FOOT AND ANKLE AND ASSOCIATED IMAGING PLANES

Structure	Location or Function	Plane
Hindfoot		
Tarsal bones	Talus and calcaneus.	Sagittal/coronal
Subtalar joint	Consists of talus as it rests on calcaneus.	
	Anterior, middle, and posterior facets.	Sagittal/coronal parallel to subtalar joint
Plantar fascia	Sheet of deep fascia on bottom of foot from calcaneus to toes, septates on its path.	Sagittal
Achilles tendon	Largest tendon of the body, connecting gastrocnemius and soleus muscle to the posterior aspect of the calcaneus.	Axial/sagittal
Peroneus tendons	Lateral group tendons from peroneus brevis and longus muscles; supports longitudinal arch.	Axial
Posterior tibial tendon	Twice diameter of FDLT; adjacent to FDLT.	Axial
Flexor digitorum longus tendon (FDLT)	Tibial side crosses diagonal on plantar aspect to insert into distal phalanges of lateral four toes (flexes and everts toes and foot).	Axial/coronal/sagittal
Deltoid ligament	Attaches medial malleolus to talus. Strongest ligament of ankle.	Axial/coronal/sagittal
Lateral calcaneal fibular ligament (LCFL)	Attaches lateral malleolus to talus and calcaneus.	Axial/coronal/sagittal
Anterior talofibular ligament (ATFL)	Lateral malleolus to neck of talus.	Axial/coronal/sagittal
Posterior talofibular ligament (PTFL)	Malleolar fossa to posterior tubercle of talus.	Axial/coronal/sagittal
Midfoot		
Tarsal bones	Navicular, cuboid, first, second, third cuneiforms.	Axial angled from true coronal plane
Lis Franc joint	Cuneiform/cuboid articulation with metatarsals.	Angle parallel to metatarsal heads in off-coronal plane
Forefoot		
Metatarsals 1–5		Axial from coronal loc., imaged with metatarsal heads in same plane

cal structures of the foot and ankle and the imaging plane in which they can be well visualized using MRI.

MR vascular imaging is being investigated as a procedure that will provide high-quality images of the arterial circulation of the foot and ankle.[22] Peripheral arterial circulation is often difficult to evaluate on patients with occlusive disease because of multiple levels of atherosclerotic disease and slow flow. The ability to visualize arterial anatomy on these patients is extremely important in planning operative management. In a small study performed by Unger et al. using 2D TOF techniques, MR vascular imaging appeared to be comparable to or better than conventional angiography for evaluating arterial circulation in the foot and ankle. With improvements in coil technology as well as other technical advancements, vascular imaging of the foot and ankle using MRI can become a valuable diagnostic tool.

Foot and ankle imaging poses a unique challenge to the operator, one that can be accomplished with precision and finesse. It is imperative that the operator have a thorough knowledge of the anatomy and most common abnormalities seen in this anatomic region so that the planes of imaging can be specifically chosen. By scanning a single limb using the appropriate coil size (e.g., quadrature extremity for the hindfoot, smallest surface coil for the forefoot), small fields of view, multiple imaging planes, and sequences that include T1, T2, and STIR, images that yield the most diagnostic information can be obtained.

References

1. Flannigan B et al: MR arthrography of the shoulder: Comparison with conventional MR imaging. *AJR* 155(4): 829–832, 1990.
2. Faulkner W Jr.: Imaging coil technology, in Woodward P, Freimarck R: *MRI for Technologists.* New York: McGraw-Hill, 1994.
3. Faulkner W Jr.: Imaging coil technology, in Woodward P, Freimarck R: *MRI for Technologists.* New York: McGraw-Hill, 1994.
4. Faulkner W Jr.: Imaging coil technology, in Woodward P, Freimarck R: *MRI for Technologists.* New York: McGraw-Hill, 1994.
5. Faulkner W Jr.: Imaging coil technology, in Woodward P, Freimarck R: *MRI for Technologists.* New York: McGraw-Hill, 1994.
6. Burk DL et al.: Rotator cuff tears: Prospective comparison of MR imaging with arthrography, sonography and surgery. *AJR* 153:87–92, 1989. Zlatkin MB et al.: Rotator cuff tears: Diagnostic performance of MR imaging. *Radiology* 172:223–229, 1989. Seeger LL et al.: Shoulder impingement syndrome: MR findings in 53 shoulders. *AJR* 150:343–347, 1988. Garneau RA et al: Glenoid labrum: Evaluation with MR imaging. *Radiology* 179(2):519–522, 1991. Legan JM et al.: Tears of the glenoid labrum: MR imaging of 88 arthroscopically confirmed cases. *Radiology,* 179(1):241–246, 1991. Seeger LL et al.: Shoulder instability: Evaluation with MR imaging. *Radiology* 168(3): 695–696, 1988.
7. Franklin PD: MR of the shoulder. *7th Annual Advances in Mid & Low Field Magnetic Resonance Imaging.* Orlando, FL, September 6–10, 1995.
8. Franklin PD. MR of the shoulder. *7th Annual Advances in Mid & Low Field Magnetic Resonance Imaging.* Orlando, FL, September 6–10, 1995.
9. Ho CP: Sports and occupational injuries of the elbow: MR imaging findings. *AJR* 164:1465–1471, 1995.
10. Franklin PD: MR of the wrist and elbow. *7th Annual Advances in Mid & Low Field Magnetic Resonance Imaging.* Orlando, FL, September 6–10, 1995.
11. Mesgarzadeh M et al: Carpal tunnel: MR imaging, part II; carpal tunnel syndrome. *Radiology* 171:749–754, 1989.
12. Franklin PD: MR of the hip. *7th Annual Advances in Mid & Low Field Magnetic Resonance Imaging.* Orlando, FL, September 6–10, 1995.
13. Wolf CR, Runge VL. Musculoskeletal system, in Runge VL: *Clinical Magnetic Resonance Imaging.* Philadelphia: Lippincott, 1990, pp. 419–428.
14. Rothschild P. MR of the hip. *4th Annual Advances in Mid & Low Field Magnetic Resonance Imaging.* San Francisco, CA, September 10–13, 1992.
15. Mitchell DG, Rao VM, Dalinka MR, et al: Femoral head avascular necrosis: Correlation of MR imaging, radiographic staging, radionuclide imaging, and clinical findings. *Radiology* 162:709–715, 1987.
16. Mayer DP: MR of the knee. *7th Annual Advances in Mid & Low Field Magnetic Resonance Imaging.* Orlando, FL, September 6–10, 1995.
17. Elster AD: *Questions and Answers in Magnetic Resonance Imaging.* St. Louis, Mosby, 1994.
18. Mayer DP: MR of the knee. *7th Annual Advances in Mid & Low Field Magnetic Resonance Imaging.* Orlando, FL, September 6–10, 1995.
19. Mayer DP: MR of the knee. *7th Annual Advances in Mid & Low Field Magnetic Resonance Imaging.* Orlando, FL, September 6–10, 1995.
20. Munk PL, Helms CA: Traumatic osteochondral diseases of the knee joint and related disorders, in Kricum, ME: *MRI of the knee.* Gaithersburg: Aspen Publications, 1992, pp. 107–126.
21. Mayer DP: MR of the foot and ankle. *7th Annual Advances in Mid & Low Field Magnetic Resonance Imaging.* Orlando, FL, September 6–10, 1995.
22. Unger EC et al.: Magnetic resonance angiography of the foot and ankle. Department of Radiology, the University of Arizona health sciences center.

18

Abdominal and Pelvic Imaging

The usefulness of MRI in abdominal and pelvic imaging is based on superior contrast resolution compared to CT imaging as well as its multiplanar imaging capabilities. These features may in fact improve accuracy in disease detection, characterization, and extent. Yet abdominal MR imaging has been plagued with artifacts caused by physiological processes such as bowel peristalsis, vascular pulsations, respiration, and flow-related enhancement. Magnetic susceptibility, often observed in pelvic regions when using gradient echo imaging with breath-hold techniques, can cause further image degradation. With the advent of fast scan imaging techniques such as fast spin echo, which enjoys temporal resolution superior to that of conventional spin echo techniques, and the use of artifact-suppression techniques there has been a significant improvement in the ability of abdominal imaging to identify abnormalities without interference from physiologic artifacts (see Fig. 18-1). Other fast scan techniques such as fast field echo, echo planar imaging, and fast inversion recovery may also dramatically affect abdominal imaging.

There are many features of MRI which render it advantageous in abdominal and pelvic imaging. MR has proved superior to CT in the detection of hepatic metastases and in tumor staging in the pelvis. Patients for whom intravenous CT contrast is contraindicated can undergo MR imaging for abdominal or pelvic evaluation. Surgical clips, which can degrade an entire CT image as a result of streaking artifacts, may merely cause a signal void in the area of the clip on MRI, with no further detrimental effect. MRI also allows organs of patients in the pediatric age group to be distinctly seen, which is difficult when using CT imaging because of the lack of fat surrounding the organs.

The characterization of fluid collections in the ab-domen and pelvis is an important benefit of using MRI because of the differences in T1-weighted signal intensity between benign and pathologic fluids. The signal intensity exhibited by a particular fluid collection can be compared to a baseline of urine, which is considered a simple benign fluid. The fluid collection can be differentiated as simple or complex (containing protein or hemorrhage), and this can be used to help in diagnosis. Tissues with short T1 times, such as fat, complex fluids containing protein, and tissues exhibiting paramagnetic effects (hemorrhage) will appear bright on a T1-weighted sequence (short TR/short TE), and will therefore appear hyperintense to urine. Simple benign fluids such as hepatic or renal cysts, which have very long T1 relaxation times, will appear dark on the same sequence and will be isointense to urine. Proteinaceous fluids actually have T1 relaxation times that are inversely related to the protein concentration. The greater the concentration, the brighter the signal on T1-weighted images. This is the reason for the gallbladder's extremely bright T1 signal intensity following a fatty meal. Both concentrated and unconcentrated bile will appear hyperintense to urine as a result of the relatively short T1 relaxation time of both. Hemorrhagic fluids will have an extremely bright signal on T1-weighted sequences when compared to urine because of blood's extremely short T1 relaxation time. This is due to its ferrous deoxyhemoglobin content, which has a paramagnetic effect.[1]

The effects of T1 shortening on complex fluids can be seen on T2-weighted images as well, especially on the first echo of a dual echo sequence. Complex fluids are hyperintense to simple benign fluids, which will be hyperintense to urine. Hemorrhagic fluids will be hyperintense to proteinaceous fluids because of their even shorter T1 relaxation time (see Fig. 18-2).

199

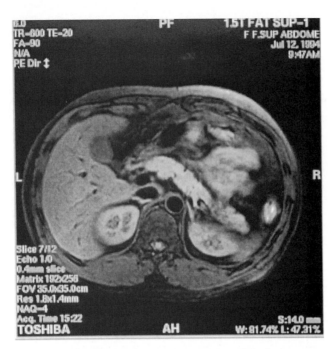

Figure 18-1 Transaxial fat-suppression abdomen image. (*Courtesy Toshiba America Medical Systems, Inc. By permission.*)

The most useful MR imaging plane in the abdomen continues to be axial. Cross orthogonal planes may be indicated when imaging the uterus (sagittal plane) or porta hepatis (coronal plane), or to better delineate tumor spread. Both T1- and T2-weighted sequences should be performed. T1 images generally provide anatomic information with little or no motion artifact as a result of the reduced imaging time. These sequences can also increase diagnostic specificity for fatty or hemorrhagic lesions that have high

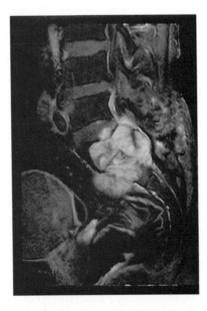

Figure 18-2 Sagittal image of pelvis. (*Courtesy Toshiba America Medical Systems, Inc. By permission.*)

relative signal intensity or for simple cystic lesions that have low relative signal intensity. Adequate T1 contrast can be obtained when the TR and TE selections at a specific field strength yield images in which tissue signal intensity from the liver is intermediate and greater than that observed in the spleen, kidneys, adrenals, or surrounding muscle. On T2-weighted images, the signal intensity of liver parenchyma is hypointense to that of fat, spleen, and pancreas, in that order. T2 images provide the best sensitivity to focal lesions of the liver or uterus and to local tumor spread. They are also useful in differentiating benign from malignant adrenal masses.[2] The improvement of fat-suppression techniques may allow better visualization of processes such as focal fatty infiltration of the liver, which usually appears as normal hepatic parenchyma on MR.[3]

The FOV selected in abdominal imaging is generally much larger than that used elsewhere in the body: usually between 30 and 40 cm when imaging the average adult. Smaller FOVs can be used when imaging the pelvis using surface or phased array coils. The larger relative size of this anatomy also allows the use of larger voxel volumes, so that slice thicknesses selected can be on the order of 5 to 10 mm, while pixel resolution can be 1 to 2 mm. This allows for an improvement in SNR.

Motion-artifact-suppression techniques prove quite beneficial and should be used without reservation. Presaturation pulses, which significantly minimize motion artifacts, can be applied in the superior and inferior directions when acquiring axial images in either the upper abdomen or the pelvis. Flow compensation can be used along with presaturation bands or can be used alone. Careful selection of phase- and frequency-encoding directions will ensure that the technique will accomplish the objective (see Chap. 12). Increased signal averaging (e.g., $N_{acq} = 8$) can be used when imaging with ultrashort TR and TE times, minimizing motion artifacts via a decrease in repetition time and improving signal. The combination of ultrashort TR and TE yields highly T1-weighted images with superb contrast sensitivity, useful for depicting lymphadenopathy or adrenal masses.[4]

Abdominal and pelvic imaging is more successful when peristalsis is minimized. This can be accomplished either by scanning the patient in a fasting state (for approximately four hours prior to the start of the scan) or by injecting glucagon immediately before pressing the "start" button.

When scanning a patient with a large abdomen, it may be useful to minimize motion by applying a compression band tightly about the abdomen or by scanning the patient in a prone orientation. Any method which minimizes the external or internal movement of the abdomen will help to produce images of high quality.

Differences in field strength can have an effect on the ability to produce high-quality MR images of the abdomen. Generally, mid-field-strength imaging outperforms high-field-strength for several reasons. Contrast discrimination suffers at high field strength because of increasing T1 values. As a result, optimization of T2 contrast is difficult because of the long TR times necessary. In addition, artifacts such as chemical shift, magnetic susceptibility, flow, motion, and eddy currents are more pronounced at high field strength. RF power deposition is also significant at high field strength, so that imaging techniques that use ultrashort TR/TE sequences and presaturation pulses are difficult to acquire owing to lack of coverage (slice decrease) and signal optimization problems. In general, however, abdominal imaging can be performed with success on a scanner of any field strength if scan parameters are optimized for the system.

MR imaging of the abdomen and pelvis is indicated for an increasing variety of clinical circumstances, which can be identified by regions of interest.

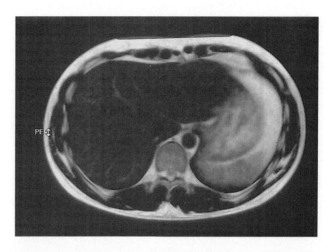

Figure 18-3 Fast spin echo T2-weighted image of liver acquired in 2 min. (*Courtesy Toshiba America Medical Systems, Inc. By permission.*)

Hepatic Imaging

Now that sequences are available that minimize motion artifacts in the upper abdomen, hepatic MR imaging has expanded. The simplest of these techniques uses spin echo technology with ultrashort TR and TE times, e.g., TR = 250 and TE = 15 (at mid-field strength), and multiple signal averages, such as N_{acq} = 8. This type of sequence provides extremely T1-weighted contrast in which almost all nonhemorrhagic focal hepatic abnormalities are hypointense relative to the normal liver parenchyma. Compared to a concomitant conventional T2-weighted sequence, in which signal intensity of the focal hepatic abnormalities is hyperintense, the T1 images display minimal motion artifacts, making this the superior imaging technique. Using fast spin echo technology, heavily T2-weighted images can be acquired in much less time, so that this technique approaches the usefulness of its T1 counterpart (see Fig. 18-3).

MRI of the liver has been recommended following other imaging techniques for evaluation of small lesions, lesions with findings suggestive of malignancy (such as ill-defined borders), and patients who have a diagnosed malignancy and an incidental finding of hemangioma. Metastases may be visible only on the MR.[5]

Imaging the liver for the presence of focal hepatic lesions often incidentally reveals a cavernous hemangioma. Liver hemangiomas, although benign with few clinical symptoms, are difficult to distinguish from other, more significant lesions on MR because of their similarity to necrotic or hemorrhagic tissues in signal intensity on T2 images. Hemangiomas generally have stagnant blood pools, which are visualized as very high signal intensity on heavily T2-weighted images. If large, they may also contain fibrotic

thrombosed areas, which are seen as relatively low signal intensity. Other imaging techniques, such as RBC scintigraphy, can also show hemangioma enhancement patterns that mimic those of other tumors, such as edematous and hypervascular tumors of large interstitial spaces.[6] For this reason, contrast-enhanced MR imaging can be used to provide valuable physiologic information and can help in benign versus malignant lesion differentiation.[7] Rapid scanning techniques can be performed immediately following the bolus injection of contrast material, resulting in improved sensitivity of detection of hepatic lesions.[8]

Recent investigation into the efficacy of MR vascular imaging of the vasculature of the liver has shown promise in evaluating hepatic and portal venous structures as well as the biliary tree (see Fig. 18-4).

Pancreas

MR imaging of the pancreas is more of an adjunct procedure. Its primary usefulness is in identifying endocrine tumors; in evaluation of pancreatitis, pancreatic pseudocysts, and pancreatic carcinoma; and in evaluation of vascular involvement of neoplasms.

Because of the oblique orientation of the pancreas across the abdominal cavity, the gland may be difficult to visualize as a whole on one slice. Identification of vascular structures relative to the head, neck, body, and tail of the pancreas can aid in delineating the gland on multiple slices. The head of the pancreas is bordered posteriorly by the inferior vena cava; the neck posteriorly by the hepatic

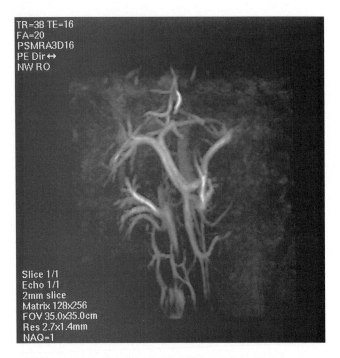

Figure 18-4 Abdominal vascular coronal image. (*Courtesy Toshiba America Medical Systems, Inc. By permission.*)

portal vein; the body posteriorly by the aorta, superior mesenteric artery, splenic artery and vein, and the renal vessels; and the tail posteriorly by the vessels of the kidney and spleen and anteriorly by the stomach.

Recent advances in fast scan imaging have allowed the visualization of the pancreas via MR cholangiopancreatography (see Fig. 18-5). The importance of this procedure lies in its ability to obtain information in a noninvasive manner, with little or no motion artifacts. Scan times are based on fast scan technology and can be as low as several seconds, making breath-hold techniques useful. Postprocessing using MIP techniques produces images that can be obtained in multiple orientations allowing visualization of the difficult to see pancreatic duct and associated structures.

Adrenal Imaging

MR imaging of the adrenal glands has proved quite successful in terms of its diagnostic capability as well as the histologic information obtained. Lesions such as adenomas, aldosteronomas, pheochromocytomas, primary carcinomas, and metastases can be readily visualized.

Characterization of adrenal lesions is accomplished using both T1- and T2-weighted imaging techniques. T2-weighted images can be used to differentiate benign from

malignant lesions of the adrenal in most cases. The signal intensity of a benign adrenal mass is characteristically low, whereas primary or metastatic tumors have a high signal. This finding will be useful in the decision concerning biopsy of the tumor. In cases where high signal intensity is seen in suspected benign conditions such as simple cysts or adrenal hemorrhage, the T1 image can be used to rule out malignancy (the T1 signal in the cyst will be low, while that in the blood will be high). In a few cases, the suspected benign mass will reveal a high or intermediate signal. The need for biopsy is then based on clinical findings.[9]

Renal Imaging

The normal pattern of the kidney is well seen using MRI, which depicts the medulla hypointense to the cortex. With prolongation of both TR and TE, as is seen with T2-weighted imaging, this differentiation is lost, as both the medulla and the cortex become hyperintense to surrounding tissues.

The primary utility of renal imaging by MR is to characterize and stage lesions. Cystic lesions can be characterized as simple cysts when low signal intensity is seen on T1-weighted images; as necrotic, infected, or malignant cysts if the T1 signal is intermediate; and as hemorrhagic

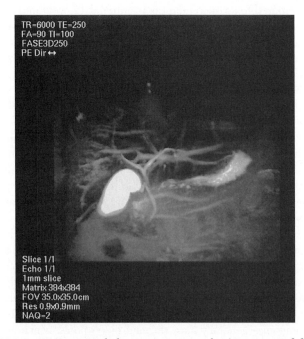

Figure 18-5 MR cholangiopancreatography. (*Courtesy Toshiba America Medical Systems, Inc. By permission.*)

cysts if high signal intensity is seen on T1-weighted images.[10] MR is used as a staging tool for renal carcinoma because of its ability to determine the origin of the mass, evaluate vascular patency, detect perihilar lymph node metastases, and evaluate tumor invasion of adjacent organs.[11] Although MR can detect hydronephrosis, ultrasound continues to be the most cost-effective method of evaluating this process. MR continues to be unreliable in the demonstration of calcifications; however, recent advances in fast scan techniques using MIP processing have showed promise in assessing the extent of stenosis or blockage of ureters as a result of renal calculi.

Lymph Nodes

Because of its high contrast resolution, MRI is a good choice for the detection of lymphadenopathy; also, unlike CT imaging, it does not require contrast enhancement. Diagnostic accuracy can be improved by imaging in multiple planes. The signal intensity of lymph nodes can be quite different depending on the T1 or T2 weightedness of the sequence. On T1-weighted images, the signal intensity of the lymph node is higher than that of skeletal muscle and lower than that of fat. On proton-density images, the signal of the node relative to that of fat is still hypointense. T2-weighted images depict nodes with higher signal intensity than skeletal muscle but isointense to fat. When T2 weighting increases, the signal intensity becomes greater than that of fat. Because of the increase in contrast differentiation between lymph nodes and fat, T1-weighted imaging is favored. Additionally, T1-weighted imaging of the lymph nodes works well because motion artifacts are decreased owing to the lower repetition times used. This may in turn allow the use of cardiac gating when mediastinal lymph anatomy is to be evaluated.

Pelvis

The ability of MRI to provide enhanced tissue contrast between pelvic structures and the implementation of phased array and improved surface coil technology has led to an increase in pelvic imaging. The zonal architecture of the prostate, uterus, cervix, and vagina can be reliably demonstrated on multiplanar T2-weighted sequences.

When this is combined with contrast enhancement, many handicaps of pelvic imaging have been overcome.

MRI is the imaging choice for staging of a variety of carcinomas of the pelvis. The choice of therapy depends in part on the size of the tumor, its location, and the invasive quality of the malignancy. MRI demonstrates these features quite readily and can also be used to assess the presence of lymphadenopathy associated with the disease.

Female Pelvis

On T1-weighted images, the uterus and cervix appear as a homogeneous signal of intermediate intensity. However, the muscular layers of the uterus and the cervix and its borders are well visualized on T2-weighted images as separate structures in both the axial and sagittal planes (see Table 18-1). Coronal imaging is generally reserved for viewing the adnexa using T2-weighted imaging.

The ovaries may also be difficult to visualize on T1-weighted images because of their location adjacent to loops of bowel and their homogeneous low to medium signal intensity. On T2-weighted images, they can be seen as hyperintense, with the follicle producing a brighter intensity than the ovarian stoma, which has a signal intensity similar to that of fat.

Imaging of the female pelvis should include axial T1- and T2-weighted images with a slice thickness that is less than 10 mm. The use of a surface coil or phased array coils can allow a reduction in the field of view so that spatial resolution can be optimized. An additional T2-weighted sequence in an opposing plane should be included in the overall protocol (see Fig. 18-6).

MRI has proved to be more effective than CT in evaluating malignant gynecologic tumor recurrences and differentiating them from fibrosis.[12] It can also be used as a reliable adjunct imaging procedure in the evaluation of congenital uterine abnormalities, leiomyomas, and adenomyosis.[13]

Contrast enhancement improves tissue characterization and has been advocated for staging of endometrial and ovarian carcinoma, evaluation of advanced cervical cancer, detection and evaluation of lymphadenopathy in equivocal cases, and for imaging patients who are unable to tolerate conventional T2 scan times.[14]

TABLE 18-1 MUSCULAR COMPONENTS OF THE UTERUS

Muscular Components	Location	T2 Signal Intensity
Myometrium	Outer	Intermediate
Junctional zone	Between myometrium and endometrium	Low
Endometrium	Inner	High

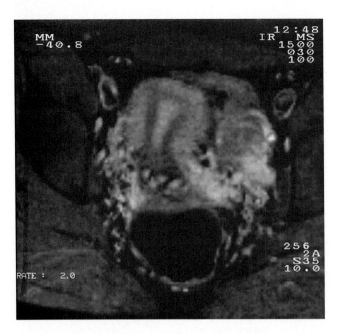

Figure 18-6   Axial STIR image of uterus.

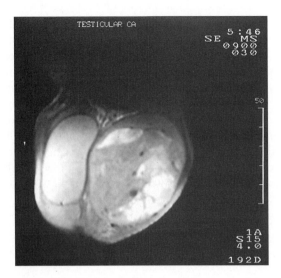

Figure 18-7   Coronal image of testicular carcinoma.

Male Pelvis

Imaging of the prostate, especially relative to staging, has become common practice using today's MR technology. Advances in coil design (endorectal coil and phased array coils) offer significant improvements in accuracy by allowing reductions in FOV. When this is combined with a slice thickness of less than 5 mm, definition of the prostate increases dramatically.

The prostate is the largest accessory gland of the male reproductive system. It is located inferior to the seminal vesicles, which lie adjacent to the inferior portion of the

bladder posteriorly. As with the uterus, parenchymal detail of the prostate is best visualized on T2-weighted axial images. The architecture of the prostate is made up of the peripheral, central, and transitional zones, which account for 75 percent, 20 percent, and 5 percent, respectively. They are all intermediate in signal intensity on T2 images; however, the central zone is somewhat hypointense to the surrounding peripheral zone (see Table 18-2). On T1-weighted images, the entire gland appears homogeneous in signal intensity.

Imaging of the scrotum continues to be performed predominantly by ultrasound. MRI may provide additional information regarding the characterization and extent of testicular masses (see Fig. 18-7).

Ongoing progress in fast scanning, fat-suppression, and artifact-suppression techniques has allowed significant improvements in MR evaluation of the abdomen and pelvis. For staging of carcinomas, MRI is the modality of choice. As an adjunct imaging procedure, it complements and enhances the diagnostic process. Its continued reliability as an established imaging procedure when others are contraindicated or equivocal is an important feature of the technology. Its use in abdominal and pelvic imaging will continue to increase with further improvements in the industry.

TABLE 18-2 COMPONENTS OF THE MALE PELVIS

Male Pelvis	Location	T2 Signal Intensity
Prostate	Inferior to seminal vesicles and bladder	Intermediate
Peripheral zone	75 percent of outer gland	Intermediate
Central zone	20 percent of outer gland	Hypointense to peripheral zone
Transitional zone	5 percent of outer gland	Intermediate
Seminal vesicles	Sagittal midline, posterior-inferior	Bright
Ductus deferens	Medial to seminal vesicles	Low

References

1. Winkler ML: Better contrast gives MR an edge in upper abdomen. *Diagnostic imaging*, August 1987.

2. Winkler ML: Better contrast gives MR an edge in upper abdomen. *Diagnostic imaging,* August 1987.

3. Winkler ML: Better contrast gives MR an edge in upper abdomen. *Diagnostic imaging,* August 1987.

4. Winkler ML: Better contrast gives MR an edge in upper abdomen. *Diagnostic imaging,* August 1987.

5. Mitchell DG: Liver: Enhancing tumors and vascular obstruction. *Diagnostic imaging,* June 1993.

6. Mitchell DG: Liver: Enhancing tumors and vascular obstruction. *Diagnostic imaging,* June 1993.

7. Mitchell DG: Liver: Enhancing tumors and vascular obstruction. *Diagnostic imaging,* June 1993.

8. Mirowitz SA et al: Dynamic gadolinium-enhanced rapid acquisition spin-echo MR imaging of the liver. *Radiology* 179:371–376, 1991.

9. Winkler ML: Better contrast gives MR an edge in upper abdomen. *Diagnostic imaging,* August 1987.

10. Winkler ML: Better contrast gives MR an edge in upper abdomen. *Diagnostic imaging,* August 1987.

11. Winkler ML: Better contrast gives MR an edge in upper abdomen. *Diagnostic imaging,* August 1987.

12. Ebner F et al: Tumor recurrence versus fibrosis in the female pelvis: Differentiation with MR imaging at 1.5 T. *Radiology* 166:333, 1988. Williams MP et al: Magnetic resonance imaging in recurrent carcinoma of the cervix. *Br J Radiol* 62:544, 1989.

13. Togashi K et al.: Enlarged uterus: Differentiation between adenomyosis and leiomyoma with MR imaging. *Radiology* 171:531–534, 1989. Mark AS et al.: Adenomyosis and leiomyoma: Differential diagnosis with MR imaging. *Radiology* 163:527–529, 1987.

14. Occhipinit K, Hricak H: Female pelvis: Overcoming hurdles to cancer staging. *Diagnostic imaging,* June 1993.

19

Cardiovascular Imaging

Magnetic resonance imaging has proved to be applicable in a wide range of cardiovascular diseases. Its suitability as a single-modality imaging tool is due to its high degree of resolution, the ability to image in three orthogonal planes as well as any obliques to those planes, dynamic and angiographic capabilities, and the ability to quantify blood flow. A unique advantage of MRI in cardiovascular diseases is the ability to identify morphology without the use of potentially harmful contrast media. This is particularly important in acute myocardial ischemia and infarction, where the heart is significantly weakened and may not be able to tolerate the added physiologic effects of ionic contrast media.

The structural detail available with MRI makes it extremely useful for evaluating a wide variety of anatomic and pathologic entities of the heart and great vessels. Some of the anatomic regions with corresponding pathologies are listed in Table 19-1.

The Heart

The heart! We all have one. It is considered a "double, self-adjusting muscular pump."[1] In its normal capacity, it keeps blood flowing to and from the lungs, perfuses our vitally functioning organs, and feeds our tissues. When it is in tip-top shape, perfusion of tissues occurs almost effortlessly. When it is out of shape, we huff and puff at the simplest of tasks. Disease of the heart is most often re-lated to overabundance of fat in our diets and to congenital heart defects. The heart is an unduplicated organ that we cannot live without.

The heart is a four-chambered, cone-shaped, hollow organ that is a little larger than a clenched fist. Two atria and two ventricles make up the chambers, each named for its side or origin. An apex, a base, and several surfaces and borders complete the structure (see Table 19-2). The heart is situated obliquely in the chest cavity, with most of its anterior surface consisting of the right ventricle.

The right side of the heart receives unoxygenated blood from venous structures and pumps it to the lungs to become freshly oxygenated. The left side of the heart receives this freshly oxygenated blood and pumps it to the aorta for distribution to the rest of the body. The "heart-beat" originates in the apex, which is formed by the tip of the left ventricle that is situated inferiorly, anteriorly, and to the left. It may be palpated deep to the left fifth intercostal space but will vary with a person's position, age, gender, and respirations. The base of the heart is opposite the apex, which derives its name from the conical shape of the heart. It is, therefore, the most superior portion of the heart, from which the ascending aorta, the pulmonary trunk, and the superior vena cava emerge.

The thickness of the muscular walls of each of the chambers is a reflection of the amount of work that chamber must accomplish. Since the atria function to move blood to the ventricles, their muscular walls are very thin. The wall of the left ventricle is approximately three times as thick as that of the right ventricle. Its workload is much greater, since this chamber must develop sufficient pressure to accomplish perfusion of all body tissues, whereas the right ventricle must move blood only the relatively short distance to the lungs.

TABLE 19-1 COMMON PATHOLOGIES SEEN IN THE CARDIOVASCULAR SYSTEM

Anatomy	Pathology
Great vessels	Aortic dissection
	Aortic aneurysms
	Pulmonary artery abnormalities
Ischemic heart disease	Acute infarction
	Aneurysm and thrombus
	Coronary bypass graft evaluation
Myocardium	1° cardiac tumors such as atrial myxoma
	Tumors with local invasion
	Metastatic invasion (e.g., lung, esophagus, or liver)
Congenital heart disease	Anomalies of arteries and veins
	Congenital absence of pericardium
Pericardial disease	Pericardial effusion
	Pericardial cyst
	Constrictive vs. restrictive pericarditis
Cardiomyopathies	Hypertrophy
	Dysfunctions
	Ventricular masses

Blood Circulation

Blood circulates through the heart by flowing from the superior and inferior vena cava to the right atrium, where it is pulled by gradient pressures to the right ventricle via the tricuspid valve. This unoxygenated blood is pumped through the semilunar pulmonary valve to the trunk of the pulmonary artery, which bifurcates to the right and left pulmonary arteries.

Oxygenation of blood occurs in the alveoli in the lungs. The freshly oxygenated blood flows through pairs of pulmonary veins to the left atrium, then continues through the bicuspid mitral valve to the left ventricle. The highly muscular left ventricle pumps blood with great force through the aortic valve to the aorta. From the ascending aorta, fresh blood is distributed to the rest of the body through capillary beds.

Arterial supply to the heart is provided by the aortic sinuses (dilations of the aorta), which bifurcate into the coronary arteries.

The coronary sinus, which is a continuation of the cardiac vein, is the largest vein draining the heart.

Heart Attacks

Heart attacks may be precipitated by insufficient blood supply to the heart muscle, which may result in severe chest pains over the area of the heart or in the left shoulder and arm. This myocardial ischemia is commonly caused by a reduction in the diameter of the lumen of a coronary artery as a result of atherosclerotic accumulations or thrombus. Circulatory insufficiency leads to local tissue destruction and causes permanent loss of muscle fibers, known as myocardial infarction. *When the damage covers a large area of the heart wall, contraction cannot take place, resulting in* cardiac arrest.

Nerve Supply

Via parasympathetic innervation, the vagus nerve slows the heart rate and reduces the force of the heart. Thoracic and cervical sympathetic ganglia evoke a "fight or flight" response, opposite to that of the vagus nerve.

The pacemaker of the heart, the SA or sinoatrial node, initiates the heartbeat. It is a collection of specialized conduction cells known as the Purkinje system. The nerve impulse is propagated over the atria, where muscular activity occurs. The atrioventricular or AV node, which is a collection of similar tissue, is located in the septal wall of the right atrium and is probably stimulated by the atrial musculature. It then conveys the impulse toward the apical potions of the ventricles by way of the atrioventricular bundle of HIS. The bundle of HIS is a strand of specialized myocardium which passes from the AV node to the interventricular septum, where it divides into right and left bundles within the septal musculature.

TABLE 19-2 BORDERS OF THE HEART

Right Border	Inferior Border	Left Border	Superior Border—The "Base"
Formed by right atrium	Formed by right ventricle and slight amount of left ventricle near apex	Formed by left ventricle and slightly by the left atrium	Formed by both atria
Slightly convex	Sharp and thin		Great vessels enter and leave here
Parallel to vena cava	Almost horizontal		

Artificial Pacemaker

An artificial heart pacing device, known as a pace-maker, is implanted and electronically activated to stimulate ventricular contraction in patients whose own hearts have lost that ability. Under fluoroscopic guidance, an electrode catheter is placed through the superior vena cava into the right ventricle, where its tip is positioned in the endocardium. A small voltage through the wire will initiate ventricular contraction.

MRI of the Heart and Great Vessels

Cross-sectional imaging of the heart provides the best overall assessment of cardiac morphology. MRI is capable of defining both anatomic and physiologic abnormalities of the cardiovascular system owing to its inherent sensitivity to tissue contrast. In addition, MRI is not invasive, does not use ionizing radiation, does not depend on body habitus or inconsistencies of operator-manipulated trans-ducers, and does not require the addition of contrast media.

Since there is a contrast variation between the walls of the heart chambers, which are signal-producing, and fast-flowing blood, which in most cases produces a signal void, an estimate of the physiologic function of the heart can be made by measuring specific changes in luminal signal to detect sites of slow or turbulent flow. Therefore, not only can anatomic relationships be assessed using MRI, but physiologic abnormalities may also be identified. Other measurable and visible structures are as follows:

- Wall thickness at all sites within the ventricle
- Coaptation of the cusps of a normal tricuspid aortic valve
- Coronary arteries at their origin and proximal portions
- Leaflets of the atrioventricular valves
- The moderator band of the right ventricle
- The papillary muscles
- The junction of the chorda tendineae cordis and papillary muscle

The MRI technologist has several challenges when imaging for the heart and great vessels:

- The heart is always in motion.
- The heart is oriented so that the long axis, a line drawn through the left ventricular apex and the aortic valve, is inferior and pointing to the patient's left.

- Flow contributes to both contrast and motion.
- Contraindications by therapeutic devices, such as pace-makers, preclude imaging many patients with heart disease.

Reconstruction of the cardiac image, in most cases, is an average of both end diastole and end systole. The challenge for the technologist is to eliminate as much cardiac motion as possible and to use scanning techniques that will enhance select cardiac cycles while slicing through the "real" axis of the heart.

Practical Aspects of MRI Imaging of the Heart

The imaging plane used to view the heart is dependent on the diagnostic information required. Standard orthogonal views may be combined with oblique views to obtain images of the anatomy that are related to the cardiac axis. Oblique views obtained parallel to the long axis of the heart as well as views perpendicular to this axis (short axis) result in added anatomic information to further enhance diagnosis (see Fig. 19-1).

Images obtained at end diastole (ED) and end systole (ES) can be used to measure ventricular stroke volume, ejection fraction, and cardiac output as well as wall thickening, by direct measurements of ED and ES volumes (see Table 19-3). Regional myocardial function can be assessed by using sophisticated tagging methods which use magnetization saturation techniques to generate planes of

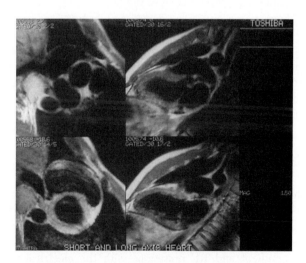

Figure 19-1   Short and long axes of the heart.

TABLE 19-3 IMAGING PLANES USED IN CARDIAC IMAGING

Information	Imaging Plane
Chamber size, shape, and position	Coronal through aortic valve at ED and ES Transverse through center of LV
Ventricular function	Three planes parallel and perpendicular to long axis of LV
Ventricular volume, ejection fraction, wall motion measurements, proximal coronary artery anatomy	Transverse or oblique sections parallel to long axis of LV at ED and ES

ED = end diastole; ES = end systole; LV = left ventricle.

intersecting areas in radial or gridlike patterns. The result is the computation of myocardial velocities at sequential phases in the cardiac cycle, which can be used to compute additional information on myocardial function.

Quantification of blood flow within the heart or great vessels can be assessed by using phase-velocity mapping techniques. Since moving spins react to the application of a gradient by acquiring a phase shift which is proportional to the spins' velocity, phase-velocity-encoded techniques can be used to compute myocardial tissue or blood flow throughout the cardiac cycle.

Cine Imaging

Several phases of the cardiac cycle can be imaged and displayed in a cine loop, much like what is done in cine angiography and nuclear cardiology. Since cardiologists are accustomed to assessing ventricular function via cine angiography, cine MRI images of the heart are especially appealing.

Image quality is dependent on the acquisition time, so that sequences must be used that minimize acquisition time as a trade-off for the acquisition of more phases of the cardiac cycle. This can usually be accomplished by using gradient echo imaging techniques and fast scan sequences.

Cardiac Gating

The heart is constantly in motion. Furthermore, it has varying flow velocities. In order to suppress motion artifacts generated by this organ during image acquisition, it is necessary to use a gating procedure that synchronizes the gradient and RF pulsations with the electrical impulses of the heart.

Gating requires that the operator link the imaging sequence to some physiologic trigger. The ECG method has been the method of choice for the procedure, since it provides the most reliable source for triggering. Peripheral gating has been tried, but problems with variability of timing between cardiac contraction and the appearance of the pulse in the periphery have been encountered.

ECG gating is complicated by two physiologic effects, both of which involve inducing an electric current that manifests as an artifact on the resultant image.

The magnetohemodynamic effect occurs because blood, which is an electrolyte solution or conductor, is moving in the presence of a magnetic field. This induces a small current, which is detected on the ECG. The magnitude of this current depends on the strength of the magnetic field, the direction of the blood flow with respect to the magnetic field, and the velocity of the moving blood.[2] Therefore, the greatest effect will be seen when blood is ejected during the QRS complex and at higher field strengths.

The second effect is caused by the induction of currents in the ECG leads as a result of the changing magnetic fields applied by the gradients. This can produce spikes in the ECG waveform, particularly T waves, which may inappropriately be used to trigger the gating function.

The problem associated with these two effects is related to the difficulty of choosing a reliable triggering point. Careful positioning of the ECG electrodes and lead wires to minimize the size of the T wave can reduce this problem. Filtering methods are commonly used to alleviate induction of currents in ECG leads.

Cardiac gating is most reliably triggered using the R-R interval. The R wave is the highest peak of the QRS complex normally found on the ECG waveform (see Fig. 19-2). The object of gating is to perform the imaging sequence during the R-R interval, when there is the least cardiac activity.

By identifying the time between R peaks, an appropriate TR time may be chosen, which will be used to acquire images. A delay time (lag time between the R wave and the first image) is usually chosen to correlate with the phase in the cardiac cycle that one wishes to identify. For

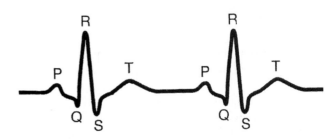

Figure 19-2 ECG waveform.

instance, to gate during systole, a delay time will be chosen that corresponds to a point during ventricular contraction, as identified by the ECG waveform, where imaging will begin. Essentially, cardiac imaging may be tailored not only to an individual's unique heart rate, but also to a particular phase during the cycle.

TABLE 19-4 DO'S AND DON'TS OF CARDIAC GATING

Do's	Don'ts
Use alcohol wipes to cleanse the area before electrode application.	Don't identify the QRS complex until the patient is relaxed, in order to reduce irregularities in the heartbeat.
Check cardiac gating equipment including fiber optics to ensure proper functioning *before* patient setup.	Don't allow cardiac leads or cables to touch the patient; RF antennae effects could result from the formation of a closed loop.
Use only electrodes that are approved by the manufacturer of your MR system.	Don't perform the gated study with the oscilloscope inside the scan room, as a skewed waveform and inaccurate readings are likely as a result of magnetic interference.
Apply electrodes to clean, hairless skin to assure close contact.	Don't use gating procedures obtained from manufacturers other than the source of your equipment.
Position electrodes according to the operator's manual for your system.	
Reduce patient anxiety before the procedure by explaining the procedure and by ensuring patient comfort.	
Use the shortest TR time possible to reduce motion; gradient echo sequences using short flip angles or newer, fast scanning techniques may be helpful.	
Use an oscilloscope to identify the ECG waveform vs. pulse identification.	

Various cardiac gating sequences may be chosen, depending on the interest of the referring physician. A data acquisition technique known as "rotational gating" allows one to obtain a programmable number of slices, where each slice will represent the heart in different phases of the cardiac cycle. To visualize one slice level of the heart through its entire cardiac phase, the cine method may be chosen.

To optimize image quality when performing cardiac gated MRI, it is important to follow very basic imaging techniques. Table 19-4 shows the "do's and don'ts" of cardiac imaging.

MR imaging of the heart and great vessels has been facilitated by advances in gating procedures and faster scanning techniques. In addition, by using conscientious patient setup procedures, cardiac imaging can result in images that are exquisite.

References

1. Moore KL: *Clinically Oriented Anatomy,* 2d ed. Baltimore: Williams & Wilkins, 1985.
2. Peshock RM: Heart and great vessels, in Stark DD, Bradley WG Jr.: *Magnetic Resonance Imaging.* St. Louis: Mosby, 1988.

Suggested Readings

Christensen JB, Telford IR: *Synopsis of Gross Anatomy.* New York: Harper & Row, 1982. Philadelphia 4th ed.

Moore KL: *Clinically Oriented Anatomy,* 2d ed. Baltimore: Williams & Wilkins, 1985.

Peshock, RM: Heart and great vessels, in Stark DD, Bradley WG Jr.: *Magnetic Resonance Imaging.* St. Louis: Mosby, 1988.

Pettigrew RI: Magnetic resonance in cardiovascular imaging, in Zaret BL, Kaufman L, Berson AS, Dunn RA: *Frontiers in Cardiovascular Imaging.* New York: Raven Press, 1993.

Index

Note: Page numbers in *italic* type refer to figures; those followed by t indicate tables.

ISBN 0-07-071801-6

9 780070 718012

90000>